Taking My Breath Away

by
Felicia Pascarella
and
Anthony Dellaripa
with
Sandy Tovray Greenberg

Order this book online at www.trafford.com
or email orders@trafford.com

Most Trafford titles are also available at major online book retailers.

Printed in Victoria, BC, Canada.

ISBN: 978-1-4269-2443-9 (sc)

Library of Congress Control Number: 2009941108

*Our mission is to efficiently provide the world's finest, most comprehensive book publishing
service, enabling every author to experience success. To find out how to publish your book, your
way, and have it available worldwide, visit us online at www.trafford.com*

Trafford rev. 2/03/2010

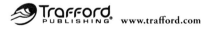 www.trafford.com

North America & international
toll-free: 1 888 232 4444 (USA & Canada)
phone: 250 383 6864 ♦ fax: 812 355 4082

This book is dedicated to everyone who has supported us and has stood by us, individually and as a couple.

Prologue

The roller coaster was about to make its second big dip when Felicia coughed and clutched my arm. Even above the roar of fellow thrill seekers screaming around me, I could tell this cough was worse than I had ever heard since we had started dating. Panicked, I looked over at her. The bright June sun made her long black hair shine, but her engaging smile was gone as her eyes widened in fear and she gasped for breath.

What if this was the "number six cough" according to her rating system? The one Felicia had talked about that day at the beach last year when she explained the rating system she made up for her coughs? She said six was the worst, the one in which she needed oxygen and an ambulance. What if this really was a six? What if she stopped breathing and died, strapped in this small car so far above the ground as I sat next to her, helpless? And what happened to being a responsible twenty-year-old who can handle Felicia's situation and take care of her?

When the ride had taken its first dip, I had laughed. Never having been on a roller coaster in my life, I had been scared to try it. Not too macho, some would say to me, but I wasn't afraid to admit my feelings. And in this case–scared was it! But Felicia, the roller coaster junkie, had assured me it was a cool experience and that I would love it. She was right, and I was glad I trusted her. After the thrill of the first dip, my fears dissolved and I was hooked. We had time to go on a few more rides before the concert started. By the time we strapped ourselves in on the fourth roller coaster, I believed I, too, was headed toward being a roller coaster junkie.

Stay calm, Anthony, I tried to convince myself. Think. Don't panic. She showed me numerous times what to do if her cough got higher than a simple number one or two, according to her rating system. Pounding her back didn't really help. Water. That's it. No, the inhaler. No, both. She always said the inhaler and water are the two things that help her the most, whichever she can grab first. The two things she always carries in her pocketbook, now in a locker in the valuables holding area.

Although this was our first time together at this amusement park, she had told me she came here all the time, rode all the roller coaster rides over and over again. What went wrong today?

If only this ride would stop. I looked at the ground, at the sky, screaming for help, only for the words to be lost in the wind–searching for any answer to this nightmare. I looked back at Felicia, who continued to gasp for breath.

Just how long can a two-minute roller coaster ride last?

Chapter One

Cough. That's pretty much what I do all day. Cough. As far back as I can remember in my nineteen years, I've never had a day when I didn't cough. An hour for that matter. Anthony, he's my boyfriend, started a slogan: "Cough for Kisses." Every time I cough, he kisses me. We've been dating for over a year, and he still kisses me every time I cough.

I get a lot of kisses.

But I am jumping ahead of my story. I have to go back and tell you about the first time Anthony called me. Actually, texted me, at midnight. Growing up together in the same small town in Connecticut, Anthony and my brother Jimmy were–and still are–best friends. I was the little sister, who hung around or tried to hang around my big brother and his cool friends. But Anthony and Jimmy went off to college, the same college, so I didn't see as much of Anthony.

When the text came, it was the end of their sophomore year at Roanoke College in Virginia and my senior year of high school. Summer had just started. The text had simple, upbeat words. *Hey! How's it going? Just want to say hi and see how you are.* No text lingo or creative cryptic spellings to decode. "You" was "you," and not "u." No signature either. The caller ID just showed up as a phone number with a local area code, but that didn't necessarily mean anything. Although the person sending me the message sounded sweet and friendly, I had no idea who she—or he—was.

I didn't mean to be rude, but I had to reply and ask, "Who is this?" Looking back on that now, how horrible I must have made Anthony feel. Yet I guess my lack of knowing who my text sender was didn't bother him. He simply wrote back and said he never signs his name because he always assumes people know who it is by the caller ID. He didn't realize he wasn't in my address book. Another ego deflator that didn't seem to ruffle Anthony, because the upshot of all this was that after two hours of writing back and forth, around two in the morning, he asked me if I wanted to go out to dinner some time.

I immediately said yes! It was very late and I was so tired, yet happy. I barely shut off my phone before my eyes closed. I had been dating someone whom I wasn't particularly happy with and had just broken off with him. From my text "conversations" with Anthony, I got to know him in a different way than just from being Jimmy's little sister. We shared movies we had seen, compared notes on what we liked and didn't like about each film, talked about people we had seen recently, filled each other in on what they were up to and said silly things to one another.

But the road to our actual first date was a little rocky. Let's just say it had to do with a girl named Emily, a former girlfriend of Anthony's, and a couple of parties where Anthony tried to avoid Emily and Emily tried to . . . . I'll get to that. But three weeks later, we finally had our first date, which led to our next date and our next date and the next . . . and somewhere in all this excitement of a new relationship, Anthony started his slogan of "Cough for Kisses."

I haven't explained why I cough a lot. I was born with cystic fibrosis.

Chapter Two

Two days after Anthony texted, still psyched that he wanted to go out with me, I got a call from him to come over Saturday night to hang out. That sounded fun, so I accepted and said I would be there right after I got off from work. At the time, I was a chef's assistant at a restaurant.

I need to define two things for you: "cystic fibrosis" and "a date." Cystic fibrosis is caused by a mutation in the gene, cystic fibrosis transmembrane conductance regulator (CFTR). By definition, cystic fibrosis is "a hereditary chronic disease of the exocrine glands, characterized by the production of viscid mucus that obstructs the pancreatic ducts and bronchi, leading to infection and fibrosis." This means so much mucus builds up in my lungs, it blocks them from functioning and I cough a lot and get a lot of infections. Or another translation: It sucks to be born with it and try to live a normal life. As of now, there is no known cure for cystic fibrosis, and it is one of the most common diseases that has a short life span.

And the definition of dating? All my friends define a date—or at least all the friends I hang around with–as two people going out together alone, one-on-one. This party came up before Anthony picked a day to go out, and being at a party with a group of kids is "hanging," and not "dating." As much as I looked forward to be alone with Anthony, hanging was OK, for now. There was definitely something going on between us after two hours of getting to know each other from our texts. I knew we'd have our official date soon enough.

I left the restaurant in my town of East Haddam, where I now live. East Haddam is located up the Connecticut River from Old Saybrook where I used to live and Anthony still lives. As I pulled into his driveway, I saw a few other cars, including Jimmy's. I entered, said hello to Jimmy, Anthony's parents, his brother Andrew, his sister Chelsea, and I patted Simon and Levi, the Dellaripa's two dogs.

I wasn't in the house more than a few minutes when the first cough came. By my second or third cough–I can't remember– Anthony jumped up and asked if I was OK. I assured him I was.

Drawing attention to myself is one of the many things on my "what I hate about cystic fibrosis" list. Actually, the list also includes saying the words *cystic fibrosis*. But then again, I don't like to substitute the word *disease* because that sounds so ominous. I know that seems weird because there are so many other diseases in the world that, while crippling, aren't as life-threatening. Disease also translates into all kinds of reactions; people sometimes even back away like they'll catch it. It's much easier to say I have cystic fibrosis, even though I've seen people also back away there, too, or if not, give me mournful looks. I feel like saying to everyone, *Could you please get educated? You can catch a cold from someone, but you can't catch cystic fibrosis.* Then I think that that's not fair of me to feel that way. If I didn't have cystic fibrosis, would I, too, back away if I knew a person had it? Anyway, I prefer to shorten cystic fibrosis to "CF," and sometimes I would like to take it one step further and simply drop the "C" and change the "F" to Felicia. I am Felicia.

Because I don't look sick from the outside, no one really

knows what's wrong with me, except for the chosen few I select to tell. Even when I go into coughing fits, most people think I have a cold or bronchitis or swallowed something the wrong way. Like the time I was visiting my cousin and we splurged on a girls' day out and decided to have our nails done. I started to cough a lot and a woman waiting for her appointment rushed over and handed me a cough drop. I smiled and nodded my thanks as I covered my mouth. Fortunately, the coughing stopped. My cousin asked why I didn't tell her I had CF. I said it could make her feel badly. A simple thank you made the woman feel good and saved me from sharing something I'd prefer not to.

CF is not isolated. CF is my life in a world that comes with its own agenda. If that means politely accepting a cough drop, then so be it. After living with CF all these years, I'm used to that.

In all the years Jimmy and Anthony have been friends, I had never been to Anthony's house. The first thing that struck me was how warm and inviting it was. The kitchen seemed to say welcome, eat, and relax. We sat around listening to music, munching on pretzels and jalapeño hummus and rehashing the previous week's *Family Guy* episode when Lois ran for mayor. A song came on with a lot of drumming. I made a casual comment about how much I adore drums.

"Really?" Anthony asked.

"Big time," I nodded enthusiastically.

Ever since I was thirteen, I've been enthralled to watch drummers in action. There's something really attractive seeing a guy play drums–the whole motion of drumming, the way a guy makes such rhythmic sounds by moving his hands up and down.

"I play an instrument."

"You do? What?"

"Drums," Anthony answered.

"You're playing me, right?"

We laughed at my accidental pun.

"No, Felicia," he winked. "I'm not playing you. They're vintage 80s pearl drums. In fact, I converted a corner of the basement into a mini disco to put me in the mood to drum."

I looked from Andrew to Chelsea to Jimmy, waiting for one of them to blow the joke and burst out laughing, but they all nodded in serious agreement with Anthony. I followed Anthony downstairs and sure enough, just like he said, there sat his drums with red, white, and blue lights draped over them and a mini disco ball hanging from the ceiling above them.

"Ta da!" He pointed to them with the same pride as a father holding his newborn baby.

Anthony sat down, gave me a sheepish smile and started to play. I was mesmerized. Yes, something about watching drummers intrigued me. And I was thrilled that even though we hardly knew each other, we already shared a mutual love of this musical instrument.

Back upstairs, the image of Anthony drumming lingered.

"Do you just do drums for fun, or are you going to do anything with that talent?"

Anthony shrugged. "You never know."

Then he mentioned he had been invited to his friend Karen's party and asked if we all wanted to go. An invitation, once again, at least in our definition, is if one person gets invited to a party, it is implied you can bring siblings or someone you are dating. At this point, I came under the category of a sibling as Jimmy's sister. What you can't do is crash a party. Everyone was in jeans and Anthony assured me the dress was casual. So that was fine. Only problem was that I smelled like garlic after spending four hours of helping to prepare lasagna, veal cacciatore and all sorts of Italian dishes! But everyone assured me it didn't matter.

Anthony, Andrew, Chelsea, Jimmy and I piled into Anthony's Honda and drove to the party. A few minutes after we got there, Anthony said he wanted to say hi to some guys.

I said fine and sat down with Chelsea. Out of the corner of my eye, I saw Emily, Anthony's ex-girlfriend, approach him. She was wearing layers of make-up, a pair of leggings, a big blue glitzy top and high heels. Totally ridiculous and totally out of place. From the way she approached Anthony and the way she was overdressed, it was clear she was up to something. Don't get me wrong. I adore dressing up–for the right occasion. Yet I don't look at clothes or the height of my shoe heel as a symbol of who I am as a person. Maybe in another setting, she would've looked cool, but not here. I overheard someone say she had crashed the party. No surprise there.

Even though Emily and I didn't go to the same high school, because I went to a Catholic all girls' high school in Middletown, a few towns north of my town, we had some friends in common. About a year ago, a group of us all ended up at a mall together. At the end of the day when Emily and I went our separate ways, we told each other that it was fun, yet neither of us pursued a friendship. Shortly after, she went off to college. I hadn't seen her since that day at the mall, and I heard from Jimmy that Anthony had been dating her. He also told me they had broken up a few months ago. Anthony never mentioned Emily in the last few days of our texts or phone calls, and I assumed he wasn't the kind of person who would date–or planned to date–more than one person at a time. I know I should have had more confidence in myself but, then again, I smelled like garlic . . . .

I leaned over to Chelsea and asked, "I heard your brother and Emily broke up, right? I mean, just wondering."

Chelsea looked at me curiously, and then assured me they were no longer together. She quickly amended her answer by emphasizing that Anthony had broken up with her. Did my face give away some emotion?

After a few minutes, the whole party decided to go outside. They passed through the area where Chelsea and I were sitting and continued on out the back door. Anthony stopped at the couch and Emily wasn't far behind. She looked like a dog on a hot day panting for water. Instead of going outside with everyone else, Anthony plunked himself down next to me. And instead of Emily moving on, she, too, stopped in front of us. I smiled politely and said hello to her but made no effort to go beyond a cordial greeting. Chelsea hopped up and said she was going outside but Emily stayed right where she was. There we were, the three of us. Anthony flung his arm around me. I got butterflies, and Emily got the nonverbal message. Although she walked away, Anthony kept his arm right where it was–which was just fine with me. More than fine!

On the way home from the party, he invited me to his Uncle Eric's annual pig roast. This time I was going as a friend of a relative–his uncle's rule.

Every year, Uncle Eric, who lives a few doors away from Anthony, has a pig roast the Sunday of Memorial weekend to kick off the summer season. Again, not a date. Although I was starting to get antsy to be alone with just Anthony–a movie, or dinner, anything–I was having fun with him, and that's how I try to live my life anyway. The more time we spent together, the more I liked him. He had a gentle way of talking and a curious mind. I loved to hear him try to figure things out. He also had a great smile and electric blue eyes. I just wished he would stop asking me if I was OK every time I coughed. I kept saying I was and he didn't need to ask. He'd say he's sorry, that it was an automatic habit. Most people are like that when they don't really know me well.

I had to work at the restaurant until ten o'clock, so I told Anthony that I'd drive myself to the pig roast. I had only been working at this restaurant for a month–and it was my very first job. A few months ago, I decided that because I was almost eighteen, getting a job would be a responsible thing to do. One of my friends worked at that restaurant and told me they were looking for help, so I went for the interview. It was my first time interviewing and I didn't really know what to expect. I thought about what I wanted the manager to know, like I am not afraid of challenges and I am a diligent person.

I also made the decision not to say anything about my CF unless asked, and then I would be honest. Although I was nervous, the interview went smoothly–and then the question came. The manager asked whether there was anything else he should know. I said I cough a lot but I am not sick–at least the kind of sick a restaurant manager would need to be concerned about. That I have cystic fibrosis. I waited for an answer and got a simple "OK." No shock. No hemming and hawing. He simply reminded me about health rules, covering my mouth, wearing gloves, changing gloves if contaminated, washing hands, and so forth. I nodded to everything he said, although I already knew all that. Used a lot of restaurant rules at home!

And then my first day came. Surprisingly, I wasn't nervous. More excited, actually. I felt responsible to be somewhere at a certain time, to sign in, and sign out. I also felt, well, typical. Now, when my friends talked about their jobs, I talked about mine.

I called Anthony as I was leaving work, and he was waiting for me when I pulled in to his driveway with my Jeep. I could hear the music and it sounded festive.

As we made our way down the driveway toward the house, Anthony took my hand–and those wonderful butterflies I got at Karen's party reappeared. This time, I actually felt my heart jump. You know the feeling. For that moment, everything in the world stops. Some days I actually wish I could freeze time. Like when I'm not coughing or not in the hospital for a "bronch," my nickname for a bronchoscopy (surgical procedure to wash the mucus out of the lungs). Or freezing the moments when I don't get asked a question about my health. *How are you feeling, Felicia? Are you still you doing your meds?* I even get asked, *How's your breathing?* Mostly, the questions are from family I might not see that often. I understand they ask out of care and concern, but sometimes I want to put a soundproof booth around me.

But life marches at a pace I don't pick, so freezing time doesn't exist any more than turning some of my dreams into reality. Like wishing I could just walk out of a hospital without a pic line. Most of my hospitalizations (especially after a bronch) require follow-up antibiotics at home that need a pic line (a tube inserted in my arm) so I can insert into it the bottle of IV antibiotics. Or wishing I didn't have to do these antibiotics five times a day for three weeks. My realities include missing special times like flying to visit my nana and papa because I was in the hospital. Or weaving my IV antibiotic dosage times into my life–or more often–weaving my life into the meds. And another reality: the high statistical probability of a short life span that CF offers, in addition to all its other complications.

Don't get me wrong. It's not as though I wake up every morning and say, "Poor me, I have CF. Poor me, I don't know how long I will live." I just wish I didn't have CF. I never slipped into being a "why me?" person. I never questioned why I have CF and still don't, or why I was the first in the family to get it. I got it and that was that. I know I can't change CF, that I can't go back to before I was born and say, "Hey, there, before you let me out of your uterus, make sure I don't have any problems." Life doesn't work like that. I don't blame anyone. My mother says I have a right to blame her–and my father. And she doesn't say that in a nasty way because they are divorced. She's just letting me know I can blame both of them. But I don't agree with her. It's not their fault. If no one in the family had CF, why would she think I could get it?

I am, however, a "what if?" person. *What if the dreaded happened and my lungs collapsed and weren't functioning? What if I just sat still, stopped breathing and my life was over?*

The what ifs? also allow me to dream, recreate my world, take me to places in my imagination. *What if I didn't get CF? What if I could go one whole day without coughing? What if I woke up one morning and somehow CF magically disappeared while I was sleeping?*

But as Anthony slipped his hand in mine, this clearly was not a moment that CF had any chance of invading my happiness.

So hand in hand, we walked to the party. It was a perfect night for a pig roast. Just warm enough to be outside, just cool enough to feel all snuggly in my favorite sweatshirt, my dad's gray *Gap* sweatshirt. As we neared the house, Anthony stopped and looked at me very seriously.

"Ah, I just want to let you know that Emily is here. I'm sorry."

I shrugged and told him I didn't care. I no longer had insecurities about Emily trumping me. I knew Anthony liked me. He said it in his eyes, his actions, the way he gently held my hand. This time I was not going to let her bother me.

"Anthony, you have nothing to apologize for."

"She just won't let it go. 'Course, we do have her to thank for one thing."

"Huh?"

"The whole reason I first texted you was because *she* had been texting me and annoying me all night while I was at the Yankees game, even though we had broken up. After the game, I was so bummed out about Emily bugging me, I wanted to talk to a girl to get her point of view, someone sensitive who could understand me, so I wouldn't feel so down on relationships. Thank goodness your name starts with an F."

"I think that comment needs a little translation," I laughed as we started to walk again.

"I scrolled down my address book, which I organize alphabetically by first names. So other than Chelsea, you were the first girl's name that popped up. How lucky was I!"

I smiled brightly as he squeezed my hand a little tighter and looked at me with a twinkle. Now, I definitely lost any insecurity about Anthony going back with Emily.

By this time, we were at his uncle's house. I couldn't believe how someone could transform a backyard into the scene that unfolded before me. I was used to big outdoor bashes, but this was intense. Huge white tents were set up everywhere. Several grills in a horseshoe arrangement were at one end of the lawn. In another corner his uncle had a makeshift platform where a band played. A beer trailer was to one side. People were in line to have their IDs checked and if not turned away, poured beer out of spigots into plastic cups. Anthony wasn't kidding when he said practically all of Old Saybrook was invited.

"This must have cost a fortune," I guessed.

"It's grown so much over the years, he now charges twenty dollars to help cover the cost for all the food and drink you want."

I reached into my pocketbook to get out my wallet.

"Oh, he doesn't charge relatives or their special friends." He winked at me. We walked on, swinging our hands. "Besides, if he did, I invited you," he added.

"OK," I answered gaily.

We immediately saw some kids from Anthony's class, so we hung out with them. I started to cough. Anthony asked if I was OK and could he do anything for me. I assured him I was fine and there was nothing to do. It was what I call a number one cough, and I didn't need water or my inhaler. Luckily, the cough stopped quickly.

In spite of my resolve not to let Emily get to me, I found myself quickly scanning the lawn looking for her. I realized this was dumb; there were at least a thousand people here. How could I possibly find her? But there she was, standing at the other end of the lawn and wearing sparkly dress-up shoes. Was she totally clueless? I noticed her staring in my direction, and I followed her eyes to guess whom? Anthony. *My* Anthony. He may not officially be mine—yet. But he certainly wasn't hers. Then she caught my eye and quickly looked away. I thought all was fine. Boy, was I ever wrong.

The band started to play a country song, not one of my favorite types of music, but the lively tune fit the whole theme of the pig roast. It was the kind of song that makes you feel like dancing to it. I spontaneously asked Anthony, only to find out he didn't dance, something I love to do. Did I really expect us to have everything in common?

So we ate roasted pig and corn on the cob, drank soda, and talked with friends. Emily was nowhere to be seen and all was "Emily" quiet–until the bonfire was about to begin at the back of the lawn.

As Anthony and I made our way there, I saw Emily walk toward the driveway. *Whew,* I thought, *she was leaving and we got through this night without any embarrassing incidents.* Suddenly, she turned around and marched directly in front of us and mouthed to Anthony, "Don't hang out with Felicia," kept on walking, and left. Neither of us said anything about this rude behavior. I figured if I talked about her, it would be as though she were still spoiling the evening for us. I sensed Anthony had the same attitude. We found a quiet spot near some trees where we could be somewhat alone yet still have a clear view of the bonfire. The warm spring day had turned into a chilly night, and we hugged for warmth and from emotion. Then the text came.

How did Emily get my cell number? I read the message. *How could you do this to a friend?* How could I do this to her? One trip to a mall a year ago and she made herself "my friend." Could she just leave us alone? Exit with class. *Friend?* Not in my definition of the word.

I read the text to Anthony, who got angry. I knew it was rude not to answer, but I also knew it would just stir up more trouble if I did. Anthony whispered to let it go and pulled me closer to watch the bonfire. Then, suddenly, I felt him lean closer and he gave me the softest, most gentle kiss on my lips. Any thoughts of Emily, nasty comments, rude texts, or CF disappeared.

Chapter Three

The day after the pig roast, Anthony and I went to the town beach. It seemed almost a repeat of the night before, as most of the "townies" gathered at this usual summer spot, with one exception. No Emily. But I was done with her. What could she do to me now? More evil looks? More nasty texts? I had other issues in my life to deal with than her immaturity. And I had the memory of Anthony's most tender kiss from last night to protect me from any of her nonsense. A-N-Y.

Jimmy was trying to get a whiffle ball game going, but Anthony said he felt like taking a walk instead. He met up with me, and with so many people there, no one really paid attention that the two of us went off by ourselves. Without saying it to one another, we seemed to have an unspoken pact that we weren't ready to declare we were a couple, sort of. Besides, we weren't really at that point.

The sun was bright against a crisp blue sky with wispy clouds, but it was still too cool to go in the water, although a lot of us, including Anthony and me, wore bathing suits. We headed west toward Harvey's Beach, a public one. We didn't go east out of respect for private beach property in that direction–like in the Fenwick section where Katharine Hepburn once lived.

I adore the beach–the soft grains of sand and the expansiveness of the water. On a clear day you can see across the Sound to Long Island. I love the smell of the salt water and air that, by the way, are good for people with CF. Salt helps break up the mucus that accumulates in the lungs and clogs them up, whether breathing it in or swimming in the ocean or a salt-water pool. It's not the magic formula to prevent anything from happening, but it does help a lot. I even have a salt-water breathing machine to access more of the benefits salt brings to CF patients.

It was low tide and we strolled barefoot along the water's edge, not talking about the fiasco of Emily's interruptions, and just enjoying each other's company. Once we were out of sight, Anthony took my hand. Again those butterflies appeared.

"I know I should probably say something to Jimmy, but I'm not ready."

I nodded, not sure what else to add. I, too, felt awkward with my brother, like I should say something to him. Walking hand in hand with Anthony was a far cry from all the times he came over to my house to see Jimmy and I tried to hang around with them. Jimmy would say, "Out of here, Sasha," his nickname for me. When he was younger, he would try to say Felicia, but it came out as "Sasha." Even though he finally was able to pronounce Felicia, he still liked the nickname "Sasha."

Anthony and I talked and talked as though we couldn't wait to know every single thing about each other. We started with my high school graduation, and Anthony asked if I was going to college. I didn't want to dwell on my CF, so I skimmed over the answer, saying I had had some rough patches with CF during high school and that my parents suggested I take time off.

"So what will you do? Take courses? Work?"

I told him about how I wake up as though each day is a new adventure and decide what I am going to do according to my mood. That I am spontaneous. I talked about possibly doing more volunteering. In the past I had helped at Habitat for Humanity. I nailed and hammered. It made me feel great because I also had the opportunity to meet the person who was moving into the house, and she was so grateful for our work. That made me want to do more. So I signed up for the Connecticut Special Olympics. We spent the day helping one mentally challenged athlete to get to all his activities on time. Those times gave me such great satisfaction because *I* was the one helping someone else.

Anthony said he hadn't any luck getting a summer job. In the past he worked at a burger and ice cream place, and one summer, he did roofing. He immediately jumped into talking about his future and what he was planning to do, whether he wanted to pursue a career in criminal justice. The more he talked, the more I realized he was just the opposite of me. He admitted that sometimes he was so busy thinking about his future, he forgot about the day he was in.

"Why don't you just concentrate on what is right in front of you? It's a really great way to live." I paused, and then added, "It's the only way I know how to live."

That discussion was so intense that we were silent for a while. The only sounds were the waves gently rolling into shore.

Suddenly, I saw a pretty shell and bent over to look at it closer. I actually had leaned over several times to examine shells. Ever since I was little, I would walk along the beach, one hand in my mother's hand and the other clutching my little pink pail that I would fill with seashells. There was something about the shapes and textures of shells that fascinated me. Today was just for admiring and not collecting. Unless, of course, I found one so out of the ordinary, I had to take it home.

"Hey, cool tattoo."

I realized that since I had on a bathing suit, Anthony saw the tattoo on my lower back.

"Oh, my rose."

"Why a rose, and what's the number sixty-five for?"

I explained how a year ago I made this decision. I loved back tattoos so I knew *where* I wanted to put it; I just didn't know *what* I wanted–definitely something meaningful and not just a tattoo for the sake of having one because it was some kind of fad. I would be graduating high school in a year and turning eighteen and thought a tattoo would make the perfect present from my parents. I wasn't sure how each of them would react when I asked. First, I'd figure out what I wanted before approaching them.

I put a lot of thought into it. What would be the most meaningful to me? One of my hobbies? My passion for animals? A filmstrip symbol to represent photography or even one of my photos? Or something inspirational? *Have courage. Be strong. Live life to its fullest.* I scratched that one. I didn't need permanent ink on my skin to remind me to do that.

I continued to think about my choices and one day, I had my answer. My mother was rearranging some boxes in the attic to make more storage space up there, and I saw the box of Christmas ornaments. Without even opening it, I thought about my favorite ornament, a fragile porcelain Santa carrying a sack with sixty-five roses inside it. Not only was this ornament very special to our family, it became the traditional gift to my teachers at the holiday season. Before Anthony could ask me why sixty-five roses were in Santa's sack, I jumped into one of my all-time favorite stories, one that I embrace with hope in my life.

"There was a woman named Mary Weiss, who had three little boys, all with CF. Can you even imagine that? Anyhow, it was back in 1965, and this mother volunteered for the Cystic Fibrosis Foundation by making phone calls to all kinds of clubs and organizations to raise money for CF research. One of her sons, Richard, who was four years old at the time, sat in the kitchen while his mother made the calls. At one point, Richard shouted out that he knew what his mother was doing, that she was working for 'sixty-five roses.' The mother looked at her son perplexed, and then realized that to him, the words, 'cystic fibrosis' sounded like 'sixty-five roses.' My mother told me how Mrs. Weiss stood in the kitchen with tears flowing down her face. That always got to me, too, because I could picture the same story happening to my mother and me. Richard's mother told the CF Foundation about this and they adopted the expression of 'sixty-five roses' as its official slogan. *Voilà!* The rose *and* the number sixty-five. Oh, and look closely, you'll see the words, 'breathe easy' that I put underneath the rose."

I stopped and bent down a little so he could see it again.

"Pretty cool, huh? A rose is the ancient symbol of love. I did it in purple because that's my favorite color."

Anthony was silent, and I got nervous that my story must have bored him.

"Anthony? You OK? I'm boring you, right?"

"No, no. I'm just blown away by the story."

"Oh."

I smiled.

He smiled.

Then all he said was that we should head back. I couldn't believe we had been walking for almost an hour. He didn't even let go of my hand as we turned around. We started back to the town beach in silence, as though we were both lost in our thoughts. Suddenly, I began to think about that day when I asked my parents if I could get a tattoo. Well, asked each of them separately.

My parents got divorced when I wasn't quite five. I lived with my mom, and my dad came up during the week to take Jimmy and me out to dinner or to go bowling or to a movie. If we had a lot of homework, he would take us to the library. He'd help us with math or research papers, and if we didn't need any help, he'd read or just sit there and be with us. On alternating weekends, we'd stay at his house. My dad always had some special events planned, maybe a museum or miniature golf. And then there were the vacations together–trips to Gettysburg; Washington, DC; Myrtle Beach. One year, my dad drove Jimmy and me to Florida so we could visit Nana and Papa. I always thought that was cool, my dad taking his children to visit his ex-wife's parents. My parents adopted a philosophy of children before divorce. After all, his ex-wife's parents were his kids' grandparents.

I was never too bothered by my parents being divorced because I got so much love from both of them. Sitting in doctors' offices with a parent on either side of me, it almost seemed as though they weren't divorced. It's not like I deluded myself that they would get back together. That much I knew. Actually, my dad remarried when I was thirteen. My mom and I would show up at my doctor's office and my dad always met us there. Always. He never missed one appointment. And later, as I got older, friends asked if they could come with me to the doctor or to the hospital, anything to support me. The doctors didn't care, nor did my parents. Through the years some of my closer friends like Kelly, my best friend from high school; or special girlfriends growing up like Daniela, Katy, Brittany, Nikki and Katelyn came with me; and boys, like Nick, who grew up in the house next to me and was my closest guy friend, or Zak and Joey, other guy friends who were like brothers. I take all my friends seriously, each adding richness to my life.

I can only remember one time when I was upset my parents were divorced. I think I was about six, so the divorce was pretty new. It was Thanksgiving, and Jimmy and I were supposed to be at my dad's but I didn't want to go. I felt sad my mother would be in the house by herself, and I cried, actually carried on rather loudly. My mother assured me she'd be fine and that I should go, yet nothing she said could convince me to do so. In the end, I stayed home with my mom and we ate our turkey together. My father wasn't even upset with me that day. He simply smiled, said, "No problem," kissed me on my forehead, and left with Jimmy.

I always appreciated how my parents handled their divorce and how they kept the interruptions to my life to a minimum. If I wanted to make plans with friends in my neighborhood and asked to stay at home rather than travel to my dad's house, he always said, "You're a kid. You're supposed to go have fun with your friends." And my mom had the same fluid flexibility. As I said, being "exes" played second place to their first priority-being parents to Jimmy and me.

When sharing stories with friends whose parents are also divorced, I hear from some how their parents aren't that willing to adapt plans based on the well-being of the kids. Like their dads never would have let them stay with their moms on a holiday. They would have insisted on sticking to a prescribed schedule rather than be as understanding as my dad, who didn't wave a divorce calendar at his six-year-old kid who was bawling her eyes out.

You might argue with me that rules are rules and life has unfair rules and we needed to learn this is the way it had to be and adults had the final say and on and on. But I could counter every one of those arguments and say my dad did the right thing that Thanksgiving and I am grateful for it.

Other than having to split holidays and special occasions between my parents, asking permission was something I had to do twice. As I got older, *I* had to do it. I couldn't engage my mother to ask my father and vice versa. I always went to my mother first. Nothing profound there, other than the simple logistics that I lived with her. More often than not, she'd say, "Go ask your father," unless it was something serious, and then she'd answer that she'd have to talk it over with him and get back to me.

So, I was turning eighteen in June and could have waited until then and not need *anyone's* permission for a tattoo, but I never thought about it in those terms. And there was no way I would get one if both didn't approve. I hate making my parents upset.

When I asked my mom about getting a tattoo, she wasn't particularly pleased with the whole idea of something written in ink on my skin that is so permanent.

I reminded her that CF is permanent, too.

My mother gave me "the look." I knew that look like the back of my hand. She'd narrow her eyes. It used to be accompanied with a comment like, *Felicia, where did you get such wisdom for such a young woman?* Now it's just "the look," and she knows I'll fill in with, *I know, Mom. Where did I get such wisdom?* I'm not sure I agree with her about the whole wisdom thing, but there are some things I feel incredibly strong about and I can be tough to persuade otherwise. I looked down at my wrist with the purple cystic fibrosis bracelet wrapped around it.

"Tell me again your design idea," she said.

"Well, a rose. And above it, 'sixty-five' and below it, the words, 'breathe easy.'"

My mom finally nodded. "How can I say no to something so meaningful? But you do need your father's permission, too."

The conversation with my dad went a little quicker. Before I even approached him, I knew it was going to result in one of two typical answers: "I'll have to talk it over with your mother," or the second, more common answer, and the one he chose this time, "Whatever your mother says."

I wasn't exactly surprised with Answer B. I assumed he stayed neutral on this issue because he had several tattoos, and it would be hypocritical for him to say no to me. My dad offered to take me for the tattoo, and my mother readily agreed to let him!

Being divorced and having me as a kid with CF could have caused a lot more problems for my parents than it actually did. There could have had been a slew of more issues, like if one parent said *yes* and the other *no*–especially, about medical decisions for me. But that never happened. I was lucky in that way. Actually, anytime I think of myself as lucky, I laugh. The joke was that when I was younger and finally understood what CF was, and that I was the first in my family to have it, I called myself "the lucky child" because I loved the irony of the sentence. Lucky and CF cannot go together.

"Here, put this away."

I was so content being with Anthony and lost in my thoughts, I didn't even realize he had bent down and picked up a shell.

It was a tiny white scalloped shell with pale orange on the bottom. I thanked him and then blurted out, "I want to take you somewhere. To my favorite restaurant. Next Monday."

As soon as the words were out of my mouth, I couldn't believe I just said them. *I* had asked *him* out. He asked me out originally, and now I'm asking him out? Most girls might trip over themselves cringing at having blurted out something so bold, and consider it lame. So unconventional. But not me . . . .

Anyhow, Anthony looked at me surprised and asked if I was for real. I nodded. He said yes and wanted to know where'd we go.

"It's a surprise, but you can dress casual."

"Oh. OK."

And that was that.

Chapter Four

It had been one long week waiting for our date, a week filled with other life-changing events–most specifically, my high school graduation. I didn't make it a big deal with Anthony because even though we had been at a couple of parties and walks on the beach, I thought it too soon to invite him to my graduation.

Monday night, when I came home from the beach, I was bursting to tell my friend Kelly that Anthony and I had an official date planned. I could have texted her, but as much as texting has its benefits, I really prefer to speak to people in person, especially when it comes to sharing something big. And this was huge.

Tuesday morning, we had graduation rehearsal. I ran into the auditorium and zoomed over to Kelly with a grin as I babbled away.

"You go, girl!" Kelly exclaimed.

She always rooted for me. Then she shared *her* exciting news and invited me to go up to New Hampshire for a week to her uncle's cottage on a lake.

Wednesday brought me one day closer to the excitement of graduating–and to my date.

Thursday night, clad in cap and gown, I graduated high school. I didn't know what kinds of emotions I would feel but quickly found out even before I finished the processional march. Overwhelming happiness equally matched overwhelming sadness. For the first time in my life, I wouldn't be going to school, yet there really was some truth to the cliché about stepping out in the world. The world I had lived in during high school had been filled with the same challenges I had in middle school, in elementary school, and the preschool years: to try to balance a life of enjoyment and fight an insidious disease. Of course, as a toddler, I didn't even know what *insidious* meant, nor could I have understood how it applied to me. I just have vague memories of watching *Sesame Street* while I sat in front of a machine with steam coming out and being told by my mother and father that this would help me to breathe.

"Felicia Anne Francis Pascarella."

I ascended the stage, received my diploma, turned to go back to my seat, and saw my mother sobbing. I knew it was about her little girl graduating high school, but something told me it was much, much more than that. Earlier, she came into the cap and gown assembly room, kissed me good luck, and whispered how blessed she was. Now, I suspected she, too, was experiencing a melting pot of emotions. Later, we'd sit on the couch, share our emotions of the day, rehash the graduation, who wore what, who said what. We'd eat pretzels, drink water, hug, and cry, just like we always did, whether I was upset or happy about something. Happy tears or sad tears. It didn't matter. We shared the moments.

I had made it through high school–four years that were like a medical seesaw. I sat with my diploma in my lap and hopscotched through a multitude of thoughts. Before my senior year, I had been in the hospital at least six times. When I ended up in the hospital in October of my senior year for a bronch, I missed one of the traditions I loved the most since freshmen year.

Every October, the entire school launches a monthlong fundraising campaign to send money to a school in Haiti. The campaign ends with a schoolwide walkathon followed by a luncheon back at the cafeteria. Each homeroom has to figure out a way to raise the money, and whichever class raises the most has the honor of leading the school for the walk. By far it was one of my favorite events. On the positive side, I told myself that at least I got to be part of the fundraising for three years. On the negative side, well . . . .

Even though I was out of the hospital and well enough to return to school a few days before the walkathon, I wasn't strong enough to do the walk. Those of us who couldn't walk–for whatever reason–stayed behind and set up for the lunch. I was totally frustrated that I hadn't raised money and couldn't participate in the walk. It was my last year of school and I wouldn't have the opportunity to do those things in that setting again. CF sucks. Ah, ha! That was the negative side.

Despite the disappointment of missing the fundraiser and walkathon, somehow, I never really worried that my health would prevent me from going to my senior prom. No what ifs? crept into my head. No, *What if I was sick and couldn't go to my senior prom*? Why, I have no idea. And it turned out I lucked out and was healthy on prom night, but I almost didn't go. I guess life can have other hurdles besides CF.

My almost missing the prom came in a way I never imagined. It was the end of March and as I said, my health was holding its own. The prom was a few weeks away at the beginning of May. Kevin, the boy I had dated all senior year, and I talked about going together but I made no formal commitment. We were starting to have petty issues, more arguments and less fun. The whole relationship was starting to unravel.

Thinking back to my hospitalization in October when I had the bronch and was so sick for a month, he didn't exactly go out of his way to be supportive. Didn't even visit me in the hospital. This made me realize that although I never expected my friends to drop everything for me because I have CF, I was lucky to have so many supportive friends. But Kevin acted as though nothing was even wrong with me.

By April, I had broken up with him, yeah, just a few weeks before the prom. Now I wasn't in the mood to go. But all my friends convinced me I should, and I finally agreed. My friend Joey was free that night, so I finally invited him, like a week before the prom.

I quickly had to find the perfect dress and, luckily, the Internet was my answer. When I laid my eyes on a gown like Belle's from *Beauty and the Beast,* I knew I had found it.

So, a date, a dress, and no health complications brought me to my high school senior prom. I was glad I listened to the advice of my friends. I had fun. This was a true live in the moment for me. I might have what iffed myself other times, and I had missed other events of the high school experience, hitting the ground hard on my seesaw, but that prom night was reserved for fun, frivolity, and forgetting anything else.

Joey drove to my house and my divorced parents, who continued to believe in parenthood before "ex-hood" stood side by side, snapping one picture after another. I looked from camera to camera as though I were on the red carpet. Then they got into one car and Joey and I got into his car and off we all went to a friend's house, where we joined a huge group of kids and the red carpet got wider as parents called out, "Look here!" and, "OK, now look here!" And we smiled and laughed and the actual prom hadn't even begun! All the cars stayed parked at this house as we boarded a party bus we had chipped in to rent for the night.

After dancing the night away, as the expression goes, the party bus drove us to a friend's house where we had more fun watching a bonfire and eating S'mores. And that was my senior prom.

Despite the challenges of these four years medically, I managed to have fun and make a lot of friends. It's funny how I tried to hide my CF for so long, but by my sophomore year, I had long abandoned that. That year, I actually did an assignment for English class and wrote an essay about growing up with CF. I only intended it for my teacher to read, but she told me it would inspire others and asked permission to share it with the class. Although I was hesitant at first, I decided helping others outweighed keeping CF to myself. At this point, most everyone knew anyhow, so did it really make that big a difference? As the teacher read the essay, I kept my head down the whole time so no one would see me cry. I could hear sniffling in the room. After that day, I was called a hero in the school and I begged people not to say that. But I realized I could make a difference in people's lives, which is why volunteering is crucial to me. So maybe some of my fellow graduates would step into their new world inspired by my words about growing up with CF from my earliest memories.

Breathing medicated steam in front of Big Bird and Oscar was a long-ago day, and as I threw my cap up in the air along with 150 other graduates, I decided my stepping out in the world would give me no more guarantees of what lay ahead than for any of the other cap throwers.

My mother, father, stepmother, and Jimmy were there to celebrate this day and all hugged me and took endless pictures.

And my friends, too, posed for pictures; we hugged; we cried; we promised to cell, e-mail, text, see each other at the reunions; and I was a high school graduate.

I spent the weekend taking pictures, reading a new book about photography, and visiting my father.

And then it was Monday. I couldn't believe we were finally on our first date.

Bill's Seafood in Westbrook, the town west of Old Saybrook, is at the top of the list when everyone talks about restaurants along the shoreline of Connecticut. You know, the kind of place where the predominance of food is fried and comes in big baskets surrounded by fries, curly or regular. The restaurant is next to Singing Bridge, which is really cool. It got its nickname because whenever a car rides over the bridge, it sounds like someone is singing a high-pitched note. There is also a dock where people can moor their boats and climb the ramp to Bill's outside patio or go inside to eat. I love sitting outside when the weather is good. As a kid I'd stand at the rail overlooking the river and toss french fries to the ducks. Actually, I still love to feed them now.

Not only is Bill's Seafood my favorite restaurant, but also Mondays are the best night to go there because a band plays jazz. So that night, Anthony and I sat inside to be near the musicians.

It was simple. I liked Anthony a lot. I liked Bill's a lot. I loved music; he loved music. I loved drums; he played drums. What a perfect place and night for a first date. If only life matched up like that.

I looked down at my outfit and was pleased with what I had chosen to wear. Around five o'clock, I had stood in front of my closet and perused my choices. I tried on one outfit after another. Skirt and tank top, black capris and white shrug, sundress. As much as I love to dress up for a special occasion, I didn't want to be too dressy, yet I didn't want a jeans motif. So I did what I usually do when I can't decide on what to wear.

I shouted downstairs, "Mom! I need you to–"

Before I finished calling her, my mother was in front of my closet, and ready to help me pick *the* outfit. Ten minutes and five outfits later, we both agreed on gray gauchos, a white tank top with two rows of small, simple sequins–but not flashy–and white flip-flops.

I knew my mom was just as excited for my date as I was–in

a mothering way. As we picked out the outfit, she talked about how happy she was that Anthony had asked me out, how she always liked him and was glad Jimmy and he were friends. I knew as soon as I left, she'd write something in her journal about the evening, or she'd wait until I came home. She told me years ago that she started keeping a journal the day she found out I had CF. It started as a documentation of my medical history but evolved into a place to try to sort out all her emotions.

I continued the whole I-asked-you-out theme by picking up Anthony at his house. I kissed my mother good-bye and she stood at the door waving as I left.

Even though Anthony doesn't live that far from the restaurant, I wouldn't tell him where we were going. The six-mile trip was fun, filled with repeated questions of, "Stop here?" or "Here?"

So there we were, sitting with our baskets filled with food that we kept forgetting to eat because we were so engrossed in learning about each other. We couldn't stop talking, I mean like a mile-a-minute-type talking. From the way we talked incessantly on our walk along the shore, I thought we wouldn't have that much left to say to one another. Maybe it was because we weren't surrounded by a group of kids at a party or in the throes of putting up a guardrail around Emily or perhaps just simply because I was so happy to be alone with Anthony and, hopefully, he felt the same.

When I think back to the evening, I actually did most of the talking, but to answer all the questions he asked about me! He wanted to know everything–my likes, dislikes, favorites, least favorites, hopes, and dreams. You name it. The one subject he didn't ask a word about was CF. I hoped it was because he didn't want to spend our first date bringing up tough issues and not because he was afraid to ask any questions other than was I OK when I coughed. I feared if he learned too much more about me, he'd run the other way. I simply wanted to have a good time and listen to the music just as I hoped he did. After all, first dates only come once in a relationship. He asked and I answered.

"Let's see. I love jazz, but you already know that. For me, there's something really soothing about it. Oh, and photography. I also love books. And jewelry. I love making bracelets and necklaces. Again, creating. Anything creative. I love to clean."

I didn't tell him that one day, I realized why I like to clean so much; that it is a way to have control over life, sort of like taking pictures and recreating what I see. Cleaning relaxes me. Whenever I'm frustrated, I polish, vacuum, and organize. Ironically, my mom installed some special and pretty sophisticated systems for keeping out dust, professional ones that hospitals use. But I find enough other things to clean in the house without having to dust.

"I love to cook, but I love baking, especially brownies, even more. Another opportunity to create–and reap the rewards in a different way as I eat them! I mean I also love carrots and broccoli, and other good foods. Oh, and animals. But you already know that," I laughed.

Some things about me just weren't going to be new information to Anthony. After all, he spent many hours hanging at my house with Jimmy. He knew I had a dog, Sasha, and used to have a bird and two snakes: Zorro, Henry and Henry II.

"And I adore photography. Oh, I said that. I love photography almost as much as roller coasters. Actually, you could say that I'm a roller coaster junkie. Can't get enough of them."

I realized I was rambling, and I wanted to know everything about him besides loving drums and hating dancing. "You?"

"Never been on one."

"Never been on a roller coaster?"

"Scared."

I gaped at him. What guy lets down his macho image to admit to being scared of anything? Anthony was really special.

Fearing I embarrassed him by staring, I quickly changed the subject and asked him what he does like.

"Besides drums? You."

"Be serious."

"I am."

He winked. Butterflies and a leaping heart. Then he paused and finally asked what I had hoped to avoid.

"How did your parents know you had CF?"

I guess I really can't separate CF and me.

"The doctors do this test for all newborns. It's called a PKU and it's to see if you had anything seriously wrong that needed to be treated right away. I think they're called metabolic disorders. Mine came back positive. Had more tests, and was diagnosed with CF, and started treatments. I was eight weeks old."

I stopped talking. I thought that was enough for him to digest and didn't want to distract us from the magical evening. I could have said more, like, interestingly, it was only the year before I was born that Hartford Hospital had added the CF screening to the PKU. Or how many people in the world have CF and that the age of the oldest known person living with CF was a man in his seventies, who ironically, lived in Connecticut. He still swims everyday. Or the interesting evolution of hospitals that once only had pediatric accommodations for CF patients are now restructuring to include more adult accommodations as the CF statistics are changing and CF patients are living longer. And volumes more, but I decided I had said enough.

He stared at me, straight into my eyes. He said softly, "I'm sorry."

I stared at him, straight into his eyes. I nodded.

Before we knew it, two hours had passed and we finally picked at our food enough to finish it. The waiter put down the bill. As

Anthony picked it up and pulled out his wallet, I snatched the bill out of his hand.

"I'm paying," I said.

"I asked you out."

"No, I asked you out," I countered.

"But I asked you out first," *he* countered.

"But I was the one who picked the restaurant and the night."

"But I am a guy."

I stared at him with an *I don't think you really want to say that to me* smirk. He sputtered. I stared some more and cocked my head in a cute way.

He put his wallet back in his pocket.

With dinner done and the tug-of-war over the bill settled, we continued to sit at the table to listen to the music. The band was about to start their second set. When they played *Fly Me to the Moon,* we simultaneously said how much we like Frank Sinatra and especially that song. Again, I asked Anthony to dance and again he reminded me that he didn't.

"I bet you're not all that bad."

"You are such an optimist."

I grabbed his hand and led him to the small floor in front of the band. We were the only ones there. If Anthony was nervous, he didn't show it. He softly took me in his arms and we started to dance slowly. OK, so we didn't exactly do what one would call dance. We swayed. Swayed and held each other close. This worked for me. If this were his version of dancing, I'd take it.

Finally, a few more couples joined us, but no one looked under the age of sixty. We were getting a lot of what I called "cute stares." I actually didn't notice at first because my eyes were only fixed on Anthony, but then I could feel someone's eyes on me. You know that feeling, when you sense you're being stared at. And trust me, I have been stared at many times, whether being the youngest couple on a dance floor, wearing my pic line for IV antibiotics, or coughing incessantly. But I just let it go.

Speaking of coughing, as the song drew to a close, I started to cough a little. Anthony whispered in my ear, asked if I was OK. I assured him that I was and gently told him that he didn't have to ask every time I coughed. I didn't want to sound like I wasn't appreciative of his concern about me, but if he continued to ask, that question would occupy a huge part of our conversations! Luckily, the coughing didn't turn into above a number one in my rating system and I didn't need water or my inhaler. All I needed to do at this moment was to "dance" with Anthony, listen to the soothing music, and think about nothing else but the sweet smell of his minty cologne and the warmth of his body next to mine.

So we swayed. He whispered into my ear that he was the luckiest guy, and I whispered into his ear that I was impressed he admitted he was scared to go on a roller coaster.

Neither of us realized the music had stopped.

After dinner we drove to Anthony's house. We lay side by side on a hammock in his back yard and gazed up at the sky. A minute or two went by as we discussed the stars and the solar system and wondered what was going on up there. I love to look for shooting stars and any moving satellites. And I always look for Orion's Belt and the Little Dipper because those are the only ones I know how to identify.

"Why do you love photography so much?"

"Where did that question come from?"

Anthony rolled on his side and leaned on his elbow, making the hammock tip a little, and we laughed.

"I don't know. I guess it's not enough for me to know what you like, but why. That way I get to know you better."

"I can tell you why I like you," I teased. More like flirted.

"I can't figure out why," he teased back. "So, just what is it about photography you like so much?"

"I guess it makes me feel good when I look through the lens. I can see what is right in front of me, yet I can recreate it. Like I have some power to change what's really there. The tree is the tree and won't change in that moment, but I can make it bigger, smaller, or wider, or look at it from any point of view I want. I've always had a camera to take pictures of friends and special times. But then I found myself eyeing things from a different angle and thinking I could take a picture and change their looks. It's a great sense of creativity. Like there was this one time when I was on a plane and–"

I started to cough and Anthony asked if I was OK. I nodded, stopped coughing, caught my breath, and again assured him I would let him know if I wasn't.

"Sorry, automatic habit," he quickly replied. "I want to do something and not just stand by."

I felt torn between simply reminding him I am OK and going into some medical explanation so he wouldn't be concerned. Tough decision on a first date with someone who gave me butterflies. I decided he didn't have to know all my CF life on a first date, but I'd share the rating system I made up a couple of years ago.

"I know. Besides, that was just a one. I rate my coughs."

"How?"

"A number one is like the cough I just had. I don't need to do anything and it stops pretty quickly. A two is when it's a little stronger and longer, and drinking water helps. Three is when water usually doesn't help, but I try it first, and then I use my inhaler. I also have asthma. Lots of people with CF do. I never go anywhere without either of them."

I patted my pocketbook that held my water, inhaler, and camera, three crucial components of my happy life. At least the materialistic components.

"Let's see, oh yeah, four. That would be a real nonstop

coughing fit, but I can tell it will eventually stop. It's when I cough and cough and cough and cough and end up sneezing and then I'm fine. It's kind of weird and annoying, and it happens at least once a day."

I hesitated before saying anything else, but I figured I started this, so I better finish it.

"Then there is a five, the kind that really takes your breath away to the point you don't know if you will, ah, um, get it back."

There was a brief silence before he asked, "You ever have one of those?"

I kept my eyes fixed on Orion's Belt and told him a shortened version of a long story.

"Only once. A few years ago. I was with my mom at her friend's beach house. Jimmy and my friend, Nick came, too, and we decided to swim out to a raft. I had no problem getting there, but on the way back I had trouble breathing. Nick slung one of my arms around his shoulder and Jimmy the other as they helped me back to shore, but I still couldn't catch my breath. Nick ran and got my mom, who raced out with my inhaler. As soon as I took a few breaths of it, I started to breathe easier. Then I sat calmly and took deep breaths on my own and I was fine. I didn't realize that because I was swimming against the current, I was pushing myself too hard and lost my breath. Now I know my physical limitations and I won't do something that puts me in danger."

I said that last statement in some hopeful attempt to assure Anthony not to be afraid to be with me. Yet I was hesitant to look at him in case he was scared, so I continued to focus on the sky. I heard his voice, soft, caring.

"So how do I help you?"

I turned and looked at him. His face matched his voice—soft, caring.

"Well, even though I don't think the water and inhaler help when I get to a five, there's always the chance, so it's better to try than . . . ."

My voice trailed off, rather than use *the* word or any synonym for it. Really, does it matter if I say die, pass away, expire, drop dead, kick the bucket? Are they not all the same?

"Anyhow, I'll go like this to say get my inhaler out of my pocketbook."

I made a motion of pointing to my pocketbook. Anthony nodded.

"And if I go like this, I need water."

Anthony nodded seriously as I pantomimed drinking out of a bottle.

"Water. Inhaler. Always in pocketbook. I can handle that. Is that it?"

I started to get nervous all over again, thinking, he's really going to freak now. I never delivered this much information to any other boy I had dated. I had glossed over my answer to Anthony's question that he asked at the beach about why I wasn't going to college, truncating the information about all my hospital visits–mostly for IV antibiotics and bronchs– during high school. At first he just nodded, and then asked what a "bronch" was. I was not used to boys asking me so many questions about my health. I didn't know how much Jimmy had told Anthony through the years and didn't want to ask how much he knew. I didn't know whether all these questions were a good or bad thing. Cared or scared? Those were the two emotions I figured he'd have. I caught myself from laughing at this lame rhyme I just made.

I felt Anthony's hand slip into mine and, again, was a little afraid to look at him, thinking I'd see eyes bugged out and a pained expression of what I needed to go through whenever I've had a bronch. To date, I have had ten of them. Plus, I hate– really hate–drawing attention to myself. Yet I had to do some explaining if we were to continue going out, which, of course, I hoped. I tried to make light of it.

"I guess there would be a six . . . if I couldn't stop coughing at all and couldn't catch my breath."

Anthony looked strange but simply nodded. "Finish your story."

"My story? Oh yeah. So my mother, Jimmy, and I were on a plane going to visit my nana. I had my tray table down and you know those little plastic cups they give you for drinks?"

"Wait. What do I do for a six?"

Once again truncation took over.

"Call an ambulance."

"OK," was all he said. I'm not sure if I traded places with Anthony, *I'd* have anything else to say other than OK.

"So the way the reading light above me was hitting this plastic cup was intriguing. I took a picture of it. It came out really cool."

"Can I see it sometime?"

"I'm kind of shy to show my work to people."

"Am I just people?" He cocked his head in this really cute way, so I knew he was only kidding. At least he was no longer focused on my cough rating system.

"Next time you're at my house, I'll show you the photo. Anyhow, my mother noticed this passion for taking pictures. One day last year, I came home from school and there was the most awesome camera sitting on my bed. She called it a 'just because gift.'"

We continued to look at the stars and I continued to be relieved he had changed the subject from my health to photography.

"Hey, did I thank you for dinner?"

"Three times at the table, four when we danced, six on the way home and in the last ten minutes, three times."

"So that's a yes, correct?"

I gently tapped his arm and giggled as a balmy breeze kicked up.

"Too bad it couldn't be summer all year," he lamented. "I hate winters on the shoreline. It's so dead here. Actually, the summers aren't always so great, so overrun with tourists, whom

I resent." Anthony sat up and gasped. "You have this serious disease and I am complaining I'm never satisfied one day of the year where I live."

"You could look at it from a different point of view. Go to Bill's in the winter. They play jazz all year round. Stuff like that. Kind of make it like summer in winter without the crowds."

Anthony looked at me with this weird expression that almost made me nervous all over again.

"You are so wise beyond your years."

"I'm not. Just a seventeen-year-old who wants to live life."

"By the way, when is your birthday?"

"Thursday."

"Like three-days-from-now Thursday?"

I nodded.

"So, can I, like, see you? Take you to dinner?"

I shrugged, nodded and coughed.

Anthony started to say, "Are you–"

He stopped himself and gave me a thumbs up. It turned out to be just a small cough that stopped right away. In that brief silence, we each stared up at the sky. Then I felt his lips on mine for a brief kiss.

"If I can't ask how you are, I'll give you a kiss every time you cough. Cough for kisses."

I wasn't going to argue with that!

"I'm afraid that's going to be a lot of kisses," I laughed. "Hold on. Does that mean I have to cough to get a kiss?"

Anthony stared deeply into my eyes, took me in his arms and lowered his lips on mine. If I thought the first kiss at the bonfire was sensual, this kiss took my breath away. He finally pulled away.

"Does that answer your question?"

I broke a cardinal rule on my date with Felicia. I let her pay. My father always taught me to pay when you take a girl out. But Felicia made a perfectly legitimate argument. She asked me on a date. Still, I didn't feel right. But how could I refuse that gorgeous smile and charming manner?

Happy, too, that I could get on a dance floor and not have a room full of people laugh at me. It was well worth it. Felicia was so easy to move around the floor with. Not exactly sure how we moved our feet, but holding her tight to me made it all feel right. And I couldn't believe we had drums in common. In fact, the whole night, we just talked and talked. She was so easy to talk to. I found myself opening up about things I'd never said before; some things I'd never even formed into real thoughts. Like when we got into an interesting discussion about how different the shoreline is in the summer compared to winter.

And then I said something so dumb about not being happy with the seasons living down here. I must have sounded like some spoiled idiot. She's got some serious stuff going on in her life and I complain about something like that. But she simply made an obvious suggestion about making summer happen in winter. I had been so blind before.

And how stupid when I said I hated the winters because it was dead around here. I shouldn't have used the word, "dead." Kind of like explaining something to a blind person and then asking, "See what I mean?" Just typical inane comments that now take on a different meaning to me. I just wasn't thinking. I'm new at this. I'll be more aware next time.

Something about Felicia makes me believe that everything in the world will be OK, no matter how bad things get. Funny, she is the one with the life-threatening illness and she inspires me that things are good.

Chapter Five

By the time dinner was over last night, Anthony knew all my hobbies and I knew his. Besides drumming being his number one love, he also was into video games and understanding the hardware of computers, how they're made—all those little teensy parts that I don't know anything about. But that didn't matter. If he loved computers, I wanted to hear all about it.

By the time we drove back to his house, we knew we had three mutual loves: drums, the beach and animals. We also knew what we didn't have in common: dancing and roller coasters. And, we couldn't be further apart on our philosophies about which part of life to live in, the now, the future or the perfect balance of the two we each needed to strive for. So I guess the quest to find that perfect balance could actually be moved to the in-common column! While I think it's good for us to have some differences, somehow I was determined to change some of Anthony's. I wanted him to learn how to appreciate the now moments and stop worrying so much about the future—and share the thrill of a roller coaster ride. Swaying could stay just as it was.

By the time I drove home, I knew I would still do my own thing each day, but I would try to look to a future more. I now had a future. I had Anthony.

Yet as I thought about some of his direct questions about CF, I slipped into my *what if?* mode. I worried about the few bits of information I had given him–that barely touched what my life was all about. Would more information eventually drive him away?

The next morning, I woke up, still reveling in the magic of our first date. Sasha climbed on my bed and wagged her tail happily, as though she knew something was different about me. My mom already knew about my date last night because we had stayed up talking about it when I came home. Actually, not talking. I babbled and she listened, smiling as I recounted each happy moment. That's the way the two of us have always been. Mother and daughter, yes, but also friends–best friends. Sometimes, people would make cute comments that we were such good friends, I should call my mother by her name, Laura. I still liked "Mom."

I sat up in bed and smiled to the air as I figured out how many minutes until my birthday and being with Anthony again. I stared at the shell he gave me a week ago when we strolled on the beach. It still occupied a special place on my bureau where I had put it as soon as I came home. I climbed out of bed, walked over to the bureau, picked up the shell, ran my fingers over the shiny surface, then placed it on the window. I kept turning it around until I was satisfied with the way the morning light hit it, then I took out my camera and clicked off about twenty pictures. Next, I turned it around to another angle and took more that way, and even more from other angles. When Anthony gave me the shell, my original idea was to make it into a necklace and wear it all the time, but I was afraid to put a hole in it to thread a chain through, for fear of breaking it. Shells are so fragile.

Jimmy knocked on my door.

"Hey, Mom says you went on a date with Anthony last night. Is she totally crazy or what?"

"I did."

"Oh." He stared for a second, turned to leave, and then turned back. "He find a summer job yet?"

I shook my head.

"Mom wants me to paint the house and do lawn work and find two friends to help. Said it could be our summer jobs. Think Anthony would be interested?"

His tone and the fact that he didn't know that his best friend didn't have a job yet told me something wasn't quite right. Anthony and I had broken an unwritten teen rule among our friends. *Never date the sibling of a friend.* I suspected Anthony hadn't said anything to him about me, and I didn't mention it to Jimmy. He wasn't home when I left for the date or returned. Anyway, this issue was between the two of them.

I nodded enthusiastically. I thought it sounded good. He shrugged and left.

I put my camera away, took a shower, and went downstairs for breakfast. Ordinarily, I'd say I did my morning routine for CF, but I was in what I called my rebellious stage. And ordinarily, my routine for CF went something like this:

I'd wake up, eat breakfast, and take my meds: two vitamins and six pills, each one with a different purpose to help with better lung function as well as one to help my liver, calcium levels, and so forth. I also have to take enzyme pills every time I eat. Two enzymes for a meal and one for a snack. The enzymes help break down the food because CF affects my digestive system.

Next I'd hook up a breathing machine for two more meds:

Pulmozyme, to thin and loosen the mucus, and *Tobramycin* (more commonly called, TOBI) that helps fight infections because infections can really make the lungs fail for people with CF. The machine has a clear tube attached to it. First, I pour the *Pulmozyme* into it, and then press a button that turns the medicine into steam, which is what I breathe in. It takes about ten to fifteen minutes for all the *Pulmozyme* to get into my body.

Before I start inhaling the steamed medicine, I put on my chest percussion vest. Chest percussions also help break up the mucus. There are different methods of chest percussions, including someone banging on your back or sides to help loosen mucus. My pulmonologist (lung doctor) encouraged that way but also prescribed daily chest percussions with the vest. This method involves putting on a vest with buckles to keep you strapped in. Like a life jacket. How ironic. I connect a flap from the vest to a flap on the percussion machine, which is rather heavy and large, almost table high. I step on a pedal to start it and it makes my body shake in its effort to loosen mucus. It's uncomfortable because it blows up (also like a life jacket) and I feel squished, and the shaking part isn't all that fun either. The time frame for the chest percussion vest is about thirty minutes.

Every day I do *Pulmozyme* and every other month I need to add TOBI to it, which takes about forty-five minutes to complete. So, on a TOBI month, not only did I have to wake up earlier to have enough time to do the extra morning routine, but also, I would have to do TOBI at night, another forty-five minutes.

Except for the enzyme pills, the rest of the day was mine, until nighttime. Then I'd take another four CF pills, do another half-hour of chest percussions wearing the vest, and if a TOBI month, I'd have to do another round of the breathing machine. At least I could incorporate the chest percussions while on the breathing machine. What a time saver!

I also use my inhaler, mostly for coughing fits but also to help me breathe a little better.

And water. I drink lots and lots of water–and not just for relieving coughing fits. I get dehydrated a lot and it's important to keep hydrated. Water also helps to thin the unwanted, thickened mucus in the lungs.

In addition to that, I also exercise because physical activity is really good for the lungs, but then again, exercise, like water and vitamins, is good for everyone. So I don't really add that to my list of things that interfere with my life. If anything, I have to hold back with exercise like with what happened that day when I was swimming and couldn't breathe. That I add to my list.

This is my daily life, or was, until my first hospitalization, when I had an infection that launched the onset of IV antibiotics, both in the hospital and once I got home.

Thus, to the already rigid regiment I have lived with since I was eight weeks old, add any posthospitalizations that required follow-up IV antibiotics through my pic line–usually for three weeks. If the hospitalization was for a bronch, those three weeks also mandated an extra dose of my breathing machine treatment for each day that I was on IV antibiotics and two TOBI treatments whether it was a TOBI month or not. To put it simply, if a posthospitalization course of IV antibiotics coincidentally fell on a TOBI month, the TOBI medicine was already being administered with one of the antibiotics anyhow and did not have to be done separately. Caught a lucky break there.

When on IV antibiotics, a nurse would come to the house once a week to change the dressing over the pic line, deliver the next week's supply of medicine, and draw blood to test various lung and other functions. At least that wasn't a separate needle being pricked into my skin because the visiting nurse could simply get the blood out through the pic line. Another lucky break.

Chapter Six

The first time I was sick enough to be hospitalized, I was eight years old and in the third grade. By then, I knew I had CF and some basics about the disease–like my lungs were different than my mother's or father's or Jimmy's. To help them get stronger, I needed to go to the doctor a lot and get help with medicine. The one basic fact I didn't know at that time was that you could die from CF. It was probably best not to know in third grade that you have a disease you can die from. That I found out in seventh grade from a boy I had a crush on. Not quite the age either–or way–to find out. But, seriously, is there ever a good way or time to hear, "Hey, Felicia, did you know that CF can kill you, possibly at an early age?"

That first time I was hospitalized, it was close to Christmas, and I had been to the pulmonologist. I was coughing more than usual and my mucus was brownish yellow, which indicated infection because it should have been lighter. As in all the other times I went to my doctor, I had to do my pulmonary function tests (PFTs). These are a group of tests where I blow into a machine that measures my air capacity, how well my lungs take in and release air and how well they move oxygen into my bloodstream. A low PFT isn't a good thing because it means my lungs are filling up with mucus, thus blocking the oxygen flow into my blood. They can also show infection, which is what I had, by the color of the mucus. My doctor prescribed oral antibiotics and told me to come back in a week to check my PFTs.

Four days later, the color of the mucus hadn't changed. I felt OK and wanted to go to school. My mother let me go but told me she was going to call the doctor. It was still pretty early in the morning and my class was doing math. I looked up from my multiplication tables and saw my mother in the doorway. She looked funny like she had been crying. Then I saw my dad holding my school bag. Why were my parents here? And why did my dad go into my cubby and take out my school bag? My parents were divorced by then, so seeing them together gave me a funny feeling, and I was frightened. Something was wrong. I didn't want anyone to see that I was scared, so I put on this huge smile. The teacher came over to me and whispered that my parents were here to take me out of school.

I dutifully followed my mother and father and didn't ask any questions except one. "We're going to the hospital, right?" I guess that was more like a statement than a question.

My mother nodded. Although I had never been in the hospital, I did know that you could get sick enough from CF that you have to go. I actually don't know how I knew this. From overhearing adults talking? From television? Kids?

My parents told me not to worry and that they would take turns staying with me. My dad would do the night shift after he got off from work and my mom, the day shift. Thinking back, I know they were saying all they could to make me less scared, but I was eight and it didn't work.

The first thing they did when I got into my hospital room was open up my little suitcase and hand me Seymour, a seal that when you press its belly, makes a barking sound like a bronchitis-type cough, much like my cough. Seymour was, and still is, my favorite stuffed animal.

My doctor came in the room. First she saw my stuffed seal on the bed next to me and asked the seal's name. I told her and then pressed his belly so she could hear him cough. She smiled and then reminded me how she gave me some pills to help make the color of the mucus get lighter but told me it didn't work. (She knew I knew the word "mucus" almost from the time I said my first word.) The doctor decided I needed some other medicine to help me. But this had to be taken in the hospital. Plus, I needed to have some medicine that would make me sleepy so she could put a special tube called a pic line in my arm to help give me the medicine in the hospital for a few days. I would also have to go home with the pic line to have the medicine for three more weeks, and that my mother would help me with it. She pointed to the inside of my elbow right where I got blood tests. A delivery of tough medical information in child-sized dosages. My doctor nodded and smiled like I should also nod and smile.

One day late in the afternoon, after my father had just arrived for the night shift, a funny thing happened. My father went in the bathroom and seconds later, a nurse walked in with a group of men. I mean, what I called "gonormous" people, who wore Hartford Wolf Pack uniforms. I didn't know much about ice hockey teams at that age but I was excited to see these men in their uniforms. Just as they surrounded my bed and started to talk to me, my father walked out of the bathroom and his jaw dropped. Let's just say he knew all about the Wolf Pack team and was a great fan. These hockey players periodically came to the hospital to visit kids and especially, more often now, because it was close to the holiday season. Later that day, I was in the activity room and the governor of Connecticut at the time, John Rowland, also came in to visit kids. I made him a turtle puppet.

I don't remember much else except a nurse who was funny and always said silly things to me that made me laugh a lot.

I couldn't wait to go home, though, because the next week my mother, Jimmy and I were flying south to visit my grandparents. Lots of aunts, uncles, and cousins were also going.

I loved visiting my nana and papa and being with my family. Every morning, Nana and I would walk along the shoreline. One of our favorite pastimes was a card game called *Frustration*. How ironic is that. We'd play it for hours. In fact, according to the prescribed rules of *Frustration*, it was possible for a game to be over too quickly, so Nana decided she would make up her own rules to make each game last longer!

Another day, late in the afternoon, my mom was still in the hospital with me and my dad came early. They stood side by side while I ate chocolate pudding. My doctor came in, saw the pudding on my tray, and asked if I liked it. She paused. My instincts must have told me if I looked at my mother, she'd be crying again. I was right. Then I was gently given the news. I couldn't go on the trip. I was too sick. I didn't want to stay in the hospital. I wanted to hug my nana and papa, walk on the beach, and play *Frustration*. I cried and cried and I didn't think the nurse who said silly things was funny anymore.

I just wanted to go home. And three days later I did leave the hospital with a new treatment to add to my daily routine– and canceled plane tickets.

Before I left the hospital, a nurse gave my parents formal instructions on how to administer the antibiotics at home. She explained a visiting nurse would come to the house once a week to check on me and remove the pic line when I was all done with antibiotics.

Now, fast forward to April 2005. I got sick. Not just sick. Not third-grade sick. Really sick. By this time, I had a new pulmonologist with a long name that started with a P. I nicknamed her Dr. P because the "P" was my last name's initial, too.

The good news is that I had no major problems for seven years after the first hospitalization. (I won't even go there about the symbolism of that number and luck.) At least, no problems that landed me in the hospital. My CF was classified as "mild lung obstruction."

What happened in '05 started out a mirror image of third grade up to a certain point before going downhill very quickly. My PFTs indicated infection. Dr. P started me on the oral antibiotic route first. The oral antibiotics didn't work. Dr. P put me in the hospital for IV antibiotics. I stayed four days. I went home with the pic line. Three weeks later a nurse came to the house to remove it. That is where the similarity stopped.

One week later, I began to cough excessively. When I went to bed that night, I could only sleep on my right side because I couldn't breathe at all if I lay on my left. I awoke the next morning with a high fever.

So it was back to the hospital where Dr. P explained that I needed a bronch. I was a little nervous, but she patiently described all the steps of the procedure. She'd insert the pic line again because I'd have to go home with IV antibiotics. After she left the room, something dawned on me. I had just finished three weeks of five doses of antibiotics a day at home. Now I'd have to start that all again.

As usual, I tried putting a positive spin on it. I'd only be in the hospital for four days. The antibiotics would only be another three weeks. The bronch would clear out my lungs. I would feel better. Besides, I wanted to feel OK for my sweet sixteen party in June. Thinking about that really made me feel better.

About two months prior to this hospitalization, around February, two major events occurred. First, my parents decided they wanted to throw me a big bash for my sixteenth birthday. Although I don't like a lot of attention on me, I never turn down an opportunity to be with all my special friends and family. And what better way than a party. My parents said they'd get a DJ and we'd dance. There was no doubt in my mind why they were making this party so elaborate, or as my father put it, a wedding without the groom.

"Can I have the DJ do the conga line?" Whenever I'm at someone's wedding reception or any special party, that's my all-time favorite thing to do. Leading a conga line would be so much fun.

Also in February sometime, I'd asked my mother for a dog. She was hesitant, believing it may not be a good idea, but she always checked out possibilities. She asked Dr. P her opinion, expecting a no. Surprisingly, Dr. P thought it was a great idea and gave my mother a list of CF-approved dogs that had hair and not fur. Within a few weeks, a Yorkshire terrier, CF-approved, came into my life. I named her Sasha, and she and I became fast friends.

Now, I hated to leave her to go to the hospital, even if it was only for four days. Jimmy promised me over and over again that he would take care of Sasha for me.

When I woke up from the anesthesia, my parents were next to me. Because I was having this special procedure, my dad took time off from work and stayed the whole first day. Dr. P came in, and I expected her to tell me that everything went fine.

Instead I got, "Let me start by saying that you don't have a tumor."

I upheld my new tradition of not looking at my mother and father when I get intense news. Dr. P reviewed what happened to me under anesthesia. When she tried to put the tube into my lungs to suck out all the mucus, a mass blocked her from getting to the left lung, so she couldn't complete the bronch. Because the mass could have been a tumor, she immediately ordered an MRI, a specialized type of imaging, to see inside the lungs while I was still under anesthesia.

"The MRI, as I said, showed no tumor," Dr. P repeated.

She paused in a strange way that made my heart skip a beat.

Something told me there was a "but" coming.

"But the mass I saw turned out to be your lung swollen shut."

Another pause by Dr. P. Eye shift to my mother. Another

to my father. Another pause. Eyes back on me in my hospital gown with a tube sticking out of my arm.

"Felicia, your left lung has partially collapsed."

I gasped, along with everyone else in the room.

With this new development in my CF, Dr. P suggested a family meeting to discuss my options. It changed the course of my CF. At this meeting I would find out what *changed* translated to.

Typically, when a patient has to make a large decision, the doctor will call in several professionals such as social workers, nurses, psychologists, and family members and friends who want to be involved. In this case, my parents, Jimmy, my grandparents, aunts and uncles, even some cousins wanted to come. And I decided to bring one of my good friends, Nikki. The meeting was scheduled for a few weeks after the bronch to allow time for all the caretakers and family members to be notified.

In those weeks between my hospitalization and this family meeting, I turned sixteen, sweet sixteen, which was also the age I became legally allowed to make my own decisions about medical care. Can you guess where this story is going?

One other event happened in that time frame. I led a conga line through the reception room, into the hallway, out the front door, back inside, through the hallway again and back in the reception room, weaving in and out of the tables, laughing the whole way. Then I blew out seventeen candles–sixteen for my age and one for good luck–and sat down to rest. I had to be careful not to overdo it because of my physical limitations.

Before the family meeting, Dr. P suggested it would be a good idea to have a short, private meeting with just my parents, Jimmy, and me, and at my request, she allowed Nikki. She wanted to give us the news privately, so we could have a little chance to digest it before telling the others. We would wait for the big meeting to discuss the pros and cons of a decision I needed to make.

Dr. P then delivered this news: I needed to get on the lung transplant waiting list.

Everyone cried except me. I don't think Dr. P's news had hit me yet. Like, she can't really mean this. And even if I wasn't numb and had processed the information and wanted to cry, I would have blinked back the tears and done anything humanly possible not to. As I got older, I hated people to see me cry. I felt embarrassed. I like to cry in my own private time.

My immediate answer was "no," a legally-allowed decision for a sixteen-year-old. As soon as I said this, everyone gaped at me. Dr. P diplomatically told me that I didn't have to give her an answer now and besides, it was time for the next meeting.

The second meeting, the big one, was a repeat of the first one except with more people crying. I still didn't cry when I heard the words again. Either I continued to be numb, was in complete denial, incredibly strong willed, or quite talented at holding back tears. At the private meeting, I had only uttered one word, "no." At this meeting, I said one less word than that.

Dr. P explained some basic facts about transplants, especially why I couldn't just have the one lung transplanted. Bacteria/infections permanently colonizing in my lungs would affect the new one, so both had to be transplanted. Then the questions flew from everyone else as I sat silently. Dr. P had already answered some in delivering her information at the onset of the meeting, but I guess it's hard to digest all that information at once. *What steps were needed to put me on the list? What could happen during the surgery itself? What were the risks? The guarantees? Statistics on survival? How long a waiting period?* I don't even remember half the questions–or answers. Someone finally asked THE question.

"And if Felicia doesn't do a lung transplant, what does that mean?"

Dr. P looked around the room with compassionate eyes, then her eyes landed on me. "Chances are she won't live past two years."

More–and louder–tears in the room. Not me. Still numb. Still mute.

Dr. P needed to give us all the options and moved on to explain an alternative: a stent. Although not as good as a lung transplant, inserting a stent would hopefully offer a viable and temporary solution. A stent could dislodge the mass, open up the blockage, keep the oxygen flowing through my body, and give me more lung capacity. But temporary was the operative word here, and the bottom line was I needed a lung transplant. I think Dr. P was giving me time to change my mind. At the end of the meeting, Dr. P told us she knew this was a difficult decision and she understood that we all had a lot to think about. She distributed pamphlets about lung transplants and stents.

As everyone left the meeting, armed with their reading material, Dr. P pulled my parents and me aside and quietly mentioned that I had one more crucial issue to deal with–a living will. With a lot of help from Dr. P and family members, I had to make decisions such as whether to implement a DNR (do not resuscitate) order and if so, under what circumstances. Tough choices.

I kissed my father good-bye, drove home in silence with my mother, Jimmy and Nikki. The rest of the day unfolded as though this meeting never took place. Not a word was uttered about it. I knew eventually this silence would be broken. It was just a question of when.

My numbness wore off that night when I went to bed. But I couldn't get to sleep. I put on my DVD to watch an episode of the *Gilmore Girls*. I have never missed an episode from the day the show started and I watched reruns incessantly. I considered my relationship with my mom to be like that of Rory's with her mom. My mom and I even made it a weekly tradition to watch every new episode. We'd curl up together on the couch with popcorn or chocolate, just like Rory and Lorelai did on the show. They had a mother/daughter relationship in which they could talk about anything–just like my mom and me. And they were friends–just like my mom and me. The only thing I never saw on the show was Rory adamantly refusing to do something that broke Lorelai's heart.

I shut off the television. In the quiet of the night, with Seymour on one side of me and Sasha on the other, the tears came and came and came–to the point I wondered, *What if they never stop?* Sasha climbed on me and licked the tears off my face. I cried more and hugged her; she licked more tears. Suddenly, I sat bolt upright; something utterly daunting dawned on me. I had been under anesthesia so I never realized the angst my parents went though, never had to wait forty-five minutes for an MRI to show whether their daughter had a tumor. How unfair for them to have gone through that. That made me cry some more. Sasha certainly had her work cut out for her that night.

I was so angry then. At first, I didn't know whom or what to direct my anger at. I started by eliminating the biggest perpetrators. Not the world, my friends, or Dr. P. I thought about when I was younger and my mother was helping me with chest percussions. She suddenly said that she could only help me to a certain extent with my CF, by talking to me, answering questions, comforting, and encouraging me. She told me another way she believed she helped me was accepting the blame for me getting CF. But I didn't blame her or anyone else. I also wasn't angry with her–or my dad. Finally, I narrowed my anger down to the medicines. Actually, anger *and* frustration that I was doing everything I was supposed to do, all those pills and all those hours of doing treatments, yet I still got this sick.

Let me say here that my parents have always been in the frontline fighting this battle for and with me. Whether a new idea, suggestion, piece of information, drug, treatment, machine, whatever, my parents have always gone into investigating mode. Nothing got past them without a thorough investigation. Plus, they were my best advocates. A favorite story my mom and I like to rehash happened when I was nine months old and in the pediatrician's office. I still went to a pediatrician in addition to a pulmonologist. That day at the pediatrician's, I was diagnosed with asthma. The doctor tried to reassure my mom and said, "A lot of CFers have asthma, too." My mother quickly told the doctor that no one was ever to refer to me as a "CFer" and to please put that on the front of my chart. She believed I deserved at least a few safe havens where I didn't get a label, and a doctor's office was one of them.

After our big family meeting with Dr. P, I launched big time into what I refer to as my rebellious stage. Not only did I refuse a lung transplant, I rebelled against all treatments: pills, breathing machine, chest vest. I only did my inhaler whenever I needed it. Oh, by the way, my rebellion didn't include my pills but did include stopping the enzymes when I ate. Not sure why. Just threw that one in in my rage.

This wasn't the first time I had rebelled against something with my CF. But the last rebellion didn't cause the pandemonium this one did. Earlier, I had protested against carrying a water bottle in school, not exactly in the same category as refusing to take meds or have a lung transplant.

I was in first grade. The classroom was different from the way my kindergarten room had been set up. There we had our own bathroom and water faucet in the room. By first grade, we needed to ask permission to leave the room to go to the bathroom or get a drink. So when I had a coughing fit or felt dehydrated, I raised my hand to leave the room. Actually, for a coughing fit, because I couldn't talk easily, the teacher smiled and pointed to the door. Yet I'd still raise my hand to get a drink when I was dehydrated. By the end of the second week of school, my teacher met with my mother and shared her concerns about how often I needed to leave the room. They came up with the idea of a water bottle. Back then, people didn't carry water bottles the way they do now. They weren't even allowed in school, so I had to get special permission to carry one.

I hated carrying that water bottle. I constantly got asked,

"How come you get to carry a water bottle and we don't?" Although I could have easily stopped the questions by saying I have CF, I didn't want to talk about it. I just said I had special permission because I coughed a lot. I remember my teacher asking me if I wanted her to say something to the kids. I told her no. I guess even at six, I didn't want to draw attention to myself. I carried that water bottle for years, and the questions did lessen as the kids got to know me, but occasionally a new kid would come into the school or someone would continue to make a fuss over it. Couldn't just let it go. But even if kids didn't ask, I'd still get looks when I took out the water bottle.

Halfway through seventh grade, I declared the end of carrying a water bottle. That I would get drinks at the fountain. My mother protested that it was important to always have a water bottle with me, so we compromised. I tucked a water bottle in my backpack, but at school, I drank from the fountain like all the other kids. But a transplant didn't come with options.

Now, with my rebellion, because all my time wasn't dedicated to treatments, I got countless hours back in my life, and on a TOBI month, I reclaimed even more hours. But, I spent all my newfound time arguing with my mother. I don't mean just arguments. I mean rip-roaring screaming and yelling matches.

Each match was the same words over and over again. The only thing that changed was who screamed louder. What we argued about switched between my refusal of a lung transplant and my rebellion against the medicines. Sometimes, after she screamed out her frustration that I could die, I'd scream back that I wanted to live *my* CF *my* way. Then it was her turn again, another argument for the transplant. Then I'd scream back even louder quoting facts about CF and lung transplants. How the lungs will most likely last only ten years, and then what? Go through it again if I was eligible? And I shouted that I'd have even more medicines. Too many for my body and my mind, for me, everything. I'd have to be on steroids for the rest of my life. Plus, there was a good chance I would reject the new lungs.

During one of the shouting matches, I actually pulled out a piece of paper with information that I read to her–about potential surgical complications such as major bleeding, pneumonia, pulmonary edema, and possibly, even painful recovery. Also, I could have the burden of taking medication that lowers my immune system response and exposes me to serious side effects that include cancer. My mother conceded that those were all good and valid points, but she argued that it also said "could" and not "definite"–that those complications were not a given.

In one argument, I told her that I believed I was given my lungs and situation for a reason and that I would rather have a full but maybe short life than spend half my day (a slight exaggeration) doing the CF routine and so forth.

She'd scream, "I know that. Even so, do you want to die in two years?"

I'd screamed louder. "I don't want to die. But I don't want a lung transplant. I keep telling you why not."

"But at least go on the list. You might change your mind. A lung transplant can give you life!"

"I have a life!"

"More life!" she screamed her rebuttal. "Why give up?"

"I'm not giving up!"

"You are!"

"Am not!"

We could never get past that last sentence. By that time, we had been reduced to playground taunting and we'd end up crying before we could get any further.

And my mother would softly say, "I'm not ready to let you go."

After one argument, after we'd both calmed down, she reminded me of when I was nine years old and I asked her if I could skip my meds.

She told me, "Don't ask me. Ask your lungs. Ask your heart and mind and listen to your body."

I did my meds!

She repeated now that she wasn't trying to force me to change my mind about the lung transplant; this decision was about *my* body and *my* lungs. She always gave me the respect she said I deserved for my choices. My mom's never been judgmental, has always had a good ear, and is a comforting person to cry with when I am upset. She was just "being a mom," as she repeatedly told me. She was only trying to make sure I saw everything clearly; that my eyes were open to what the world and what my choice now could mean to me later. Isn't that one of a parent's role?

Deep down, I knew all these arguments were more about my parents' fear of losing me than being angry. Both of them had always valued my opinion about my own disease. But this wasn't about value or respect. All the fighting stemmed from fear, on both our parts. I saw the frustration, pain and helplessness in her, and each of these emotions brought me such sadness. She *was* just being a mom. So how could I hurt her so much? What if the roles were reversed? What if I were my mother–a loving, give-up-the-world-for-my-child-type mother, a mirror image of my mother–and my child screamed at me that she wouldn't do something to prolong a challenged lifespan? No wonder my mom fought me so hard about this. My heart broke for her.

Eventually, the fights about the lung transplant were shorter, not quieter or less painful. Just shorter.

"Felicia, why won't you–" she shouted.

"Mom, no!" I'd shout equally as loud.

Finally, I put a moratorium on any mention of a lung transplant and to this no-win situation. I couldn't tear up my mother like this any more, and I decided that if I only had two years to live, I didn't want to spend them fighting about why I wouldn't do my meds or have a lung transplant.

My mother agreed to my terms to stop trying to talk me into a lung transplant but reserved the right to continue to ask why. She vowed she'd never give up asking me that question. Thus, her concession was to be allowed to ask why whenever she wanted; my concession was I didn't have to answer.

Laura's Journal

A year after Felicia was born and diagnosed with CF, I started down a path determined to find ways to teach her and me how people live with a fatal disease. I went to a workshop by Dr. Bernie Siegel (the doctor who wrote *Love, Medicine and Miracles)*. There, a middle-aged man stood up and shared that his wife, who was sitting beside him, decided to stop her chemotherapy. The husband didn't agree that this was the right decision. Dr. Siegel said it was his *wife's* disease and *her* choice. In that moment I realized the day would come when I would have to hand over the reins of this disease to Felicia. Yet as a parent, I have found one of the most challenging things I need to do is to let my children be who they are and not what I think they should be. That challenge was really put to the test with Felicia's decision.

I spent my daughter's first fifteen years on this Earth trying to control the uncontrollable by keeping her environment clean, keeping sick family members and friends away from her, singing *If I Were a Rich Man* over and over again so she would do her meds, so that her lungs would be in good condition for when they found a cure. It felt like I was chasing a train for fifteen years, and when we found out how bad her lung was, that train went out of sight along with the hope that a cure would help her. Since then, it has truly been one day at a time, knowing the future is not in my hands. Was it the time to hand over the reins?

Now, I've exhausted my arguments with Felicia about the lung transplant. She has been adamant about her decision. I asked her, "Don't you want to learn to drive? Be in love? Marry? Make love?" Her answers were no to all of the above. Perhaps, at this stage of her life, she was satisfied with all she'd experienced, felt and loved. As an adult, I couldn't fathom not wanting more in, and from, life, but somewhere in our screaming, she did teach me the freedom that comes when one accepts without the need to add or alter. I got so desperate over the lung transplant, I even threw her a life jacket. Gave her the choice to chuck all her meds, leave school, and travel around the world, but she wanted to stay in school. She said she'd travel during holidays. At least one of us made a mature decision!

I can't imagine the unimaginable of saying good-bye to her, to my precious daughter–my young baby with an old soul–to someone I love deeply as I do Jimmy, so I try to focus on this day and all the days we have had.

Yet perhaps this was the time I had to turn over the reins, as I had learned at that workshop with Dr. Siegel. But I wasn't ready.

That first morning after my mother and I agreed to our terms, I came down to breakfast, bypassed the breathing machine and chest vest patiently waiting for me. After my mother kissed me good morning, she nodded toward my breathing machine. My mother kept her end of the bargain by not saying anything. But in forming our no-mention-of-meds-and-transplant treaty, nothing was ever said about nonverbal communication–the sad eyes, pained expressions, and hopeful nods toward the abandoned breathing equipment in the corner of the kitchen. I never amended the agreement to eliminate looks. How much more could I hurt her?

And where was my father in all these fights? From the moment he heard the news and my refusal, he echoed my mother's torment about my decision. The difference was that my dad and I skipped the arguments. He just asked why. All the time. Just like my mom. It saddened me just as much to hurt my dad. It was different living with my mother because I saw the pain on her face every day. I could pretend my father still had a smile on his face–until he came up during the week to see me or I went to his house. No more pretending then.

And Jimmy. If he were in the room when an argument broke out, he'd head to his bedroom and shut the door. Something he'd done when he was upset ever since he was little. Once or twice, he'd stop by my room and would say, "Hey, Sasha, maybe a transplant wasn't so bad."

I knew he felt awful, the sibling without the CF.

It wasn't only my mother, father, and Jimmy. Nana, Papa, my other grandparents, stepmother, aunts, uncles, cousins, and even friends asked basically the same question or gave advice in various forms. *Don't you want to be on the list, Felicia? Just in case, Felicia. At least the inactive list, Felicia. You have that option if you change your mind, Felicia. You know, Felicia, if I needed a transplant for my lung problem, I'd do it.*

That last comment was from Nana, which hurt in a different way than the others. Stung extra hard. When I was nine years old (the year after my first hospitalization in third grade), my nana was diagnosed with emphysema. She never allowed that to get in the way of us having fun. Because of her emphysema, Nana needed to do breathing machine treatments, too. Whenever we visited, we never did them together. I'd do my treatment in my room and she'd do her treatment in hers. As close as we were, we didn't share that time together. But she always asked, "I did my machine. Did you do yours?"

I would later understand about genetics. Both parents have to be carriers of the CF gene. And my Nana had the genetic screening and was a carrier. One of my grandparents on my dad's side also had to be a carrier. That was, to date, as much as science knows. Carriers do not have health issues, so Nana's health issues had nothing to do with me having CF. But hurting her about my transplant decision came with different parameters.

And Dr. P? Just as I wanted to please my friends and family, it was equally important to me to please her. She meant more to me than just being my pulmonologist; she was an integral part of my life on so many levels. I knew she couldn't force me into anything legally, but I also knew she was fighting for my life to the fullest and trying to provide the best for me. So as I shook my head to her, too, I knew that I disappointed most of the people closest to me.

One common plea from all those involved was at least to talk to someone who had had a transplant, but that whole thing about meeting someone else with CF and talking and comparing was just not me. If someone wanted to meet me and ask for help or a question I would, but not the other way around. So another "no" got added to the list.

I did concede to one plea–to talk to a psychologist–but I only went to one session and chose not to go back. My answer stayed the same.

It hurt to hurt my doctor and everyone else, but, then again, it was my life. So whom do I make happy?

Each morning of my treatment boycott brought an intense sense of freedom as I woke up at a more tolerable hour and took pleasure in the fact that I had all those minutes back to me. I expected the feeling to wear off after a few days. It didn't.

Then the strangest thing happened. About a year after I launched my anti-meds campaign, I woke up one morning and decided to do my treatment and complete each part in full. All of it–breathing machine, chest percussions . . . . I wish I could tell you I had some epiphany about the importance of taking medicines, being committed to the premise that it was the right thing to do, the responsible thing to take care of myself, or maturing. I could take it deeper and conjecture all sorts of reasons like maybe everyone was right. Or my body subconsciously told me to do so, or, if not my body, my soul. But I didn't have any heroic revelation. I made the decision with the same spontaneity as when I decide whether to plant flowers on a given day, make a piece of jewelry, or shoot off a round of pictures.

I entered the kitchen, ate breakfast and swallowed each pill. I hooked up my breathing machine, poured in the medicine, put on my chest percussion vest, buckled myself in, pressed the pedal, shook, and breathed in medicated steam. My mother never said a word, just looked at me and gave me a smile. It's amazing how much a smile can say.

And just as my spontaneous, "unprofound" reason for waving the white flag and reinstating my CF routine, so, too, would a day come when I would wake up and declare another rebellion with no reason other than I simply didn't want to do it. It takes too much time.

By the time Anthony came in my life, I had a reputation with my doctor for not following her orders. I was also back to a rebel phase then. Besides, the stent, which was supposed to be a temporary solution for a few weeks, turned in to two years and still seemed to work–for the time being. My PFTs kept coming back fine, and I had no reactions to the stent, so Dr. P didn't want to risk taking it out.

So I am a confusing person. Just as CF is a complicated disease and no two cases are exactly alike–because CF can affect so many parts of the body–so too are my emotions. Of course I didn't want to die. And, of course a lung transplant could have given me a longer life. But each decision comes with attachments. A new lung could only give me maybe ten years max, and then what? There may not be a "then what?" other than hopes and prayers. So if I can prolong having a transplant, when and if I do, the time it buys me can give me even a longer life. Or that might not be the answer. It is not a square in a square, one of Anthony's favorite expressions.

So I did survive beyond the estimated two years. Do I think Dr. P didn't know what she was talking about? No. I believe in her knowledge and trust her assessment of my situation. Do I believe in miracles? Faith? Higher power? I, the mightier one? Or something or someone out there I have no idea what name to call? I know my parents always encouraged me to ask a lot of questions, research, learn, and find the perfect balance between listening to others and taking charge of my own health. When I was little, taking charge was more someone else's doing, but as I got older, I gained the confidence to be my own person. Yet I doubt anyone ever expected me to say no to a lung transplant. Like I said, complicated and confusing–the disease and me.

After the surgery to have the stent inserted, when I was well enough to go out, a traveling carnival was in town. My mother suggested we go and also suggested I invite a friend. That day, my friend Hannah from the neighborhood, my mother, and I walked around looking at the rides, eating hot buttered popcorn. I walked a bit slowly, of course, because I was still recuperating. And part of recuperating was a pic line, the antibiotics–you know the drill. I asked my mom if I could go on a ride and she agreed, but the only one tame enough was a little Ferris wheel. No roller coaster ride for me that day. My mom pointed to a picnic table near the ride and said she'd wait for us there and to come right back after it was over. I think she was nervous.

Hannah and I stood in line. When it was our turn to give the tickets to the man running the ride, he stared at the pic line sticking out of my arm like he had just seen King Kong, but he didn't say anything. As he stood next to the car while we climbed in, he stared again at the pic line, and asked, "Are you sure you're OK? I mean, you're not going to die on this?"

I nodded, yet he still looked skeptical. The ride started up and it felt so good to feel the wind in my face, to laugh and be normal, whatever definition of normal I could apply to my life. But suddenly, we were back at the beginning and the car stopped and the man loudly announced that the ride was over. Hannah and I looked at each other shocked. Let's just say it was the shortest ferris wheel ride I ever had been on. We didn't say anything to the man and got off to find my mom, giggling uncontrollably as we recounted the story.

Laura's Journal

> Letting Felicia take that ferris wheel ride was a milestone in her life. It was her first time in public–out in the world–with a pic line. I waited nervously for the two girls to finish the ride, and when Felicia laughed hysterically about the man who was afraid to let her on the ride, I knew that combining antibiotics and life was doable. She could have been the kind of kid who got angry with the man, argued with him, frustrated that he stopped the ride early. Instead, she turned it into a humorous adventure, a story to retell, each time giggling about it just as much as the first time. That day I knew she would approach life with the zeal she always has despite the obstacles. It was her milestone that day, but mine as well.

Back to the morning after my first date with Anthony. Still giddy, and still in the throes of a rebellious stage, I entered the kitchen, swallowed my pills and ate some cereal, the entire time keeping my head lowered. Then I told my mother I was going to take some pictures in the garden.

I could never look directly at my mother when I was supposed to be doing my treatment but wasn't. I couldn't take the ever-present pained expression I'd see in her eyes, the sadness in her face, and the body language that also spoke of heartbreak. That was the worst part of my rebellious streak. I wished I could rebel *and* have my mother's approval, but that would no more happen than using the words "lucky child" and "CF" in the same sentence.

Just as I finished my cereal and was rinsing the bowl, my cell phone rang. Anthony wanted to go to the movies that night.

"Tonight? But, I thought you said you'd see me Thursday for my birthday."

"I did."

Silence.

"I don't want to wait until Thursday to see you."

Silence.

"What time should I be ready?" I asked.

I turned to my mother and told her I was going to the movies that night. She smiled, nodded toward the abandoned breathing machine, and asked, "Why, Felicia, honey, why?"

Because our agreement still mandated that she could always ask why and I could always refuse to answer, I kissed her, grabbed my camera with its telephoto lens, and slipped outside into the garden to recreate what I saw.

Anthony and I stood in line to get our tickets. As we got to the cashier, Anthony started to say, "Two adults for–" and before he finished saying which movie, I coughed. He turned, gave me a quick kiss on my cheek, turned back to the cashier, and said, "Ah, for *Shrek 3*."

The cashier looked at Anthony puzzled, shrugged, and said, "That'll be $18.00."

If he only knew.

Anthony already had a twenty-dollar bill in his hand, which he quickly handed to the cashier and winked at me.

"Want anything?"

"Can you see if they have Sour Patch Kids? They're my favorite."

We sat in the darkened theater and held hands. Occasionally, I'd lay my head on his shoulder. When something funny happened and we laughed, we looked at each other. Like a common connection.

At one point, I was staring at one of my candies a little longer because in the darkened theater, I couldn't tell if it was red or orange. Anthony leaned over and whispered, "What are you doing?" I explained that I only liked the red and the green ones.

"Oh," was all he said and turned his attention back to the movie.

After I finished all the red and the green ones, I handed him the bag and asked if he wanted the rest. He polished off the other colors.

On the way out of the theater, Anthony tossed the empty bag in the trashcan and asked me what I usually did with all the other colors left in the bag. I told him that Jimmy ate them.

Chapter Seven

Finally, my eighteenth birthday arrived and I couldn't contain my excitement. I knew Anthony had something planned for me but he wouldn't give me one clue. All he said was to dress up and be ready at six. He had no idea at the time that I didn't like surprises. I like surprising people, but I'd rather know what was coming my way. I didn't tell him this, though. I could probably go into some deep philosophical explanation here about why I'm like this and somehow make a connection to CF, but I have no idea why I feel that way about surprises and leave it at that. Not everything in my life has to be attached at the hip to CF.

The day started with not a surprise, but a tradition I look forward to every year. Each birthday, Jimmy's and mine, my mother decorates the whole first floor of the house with streamers, banners and balloons. And she always leaves it up for two weeks, to keep the celebration going. I woke up and bolted out of bed, rushed downstairs, like I do on Christmas morning. I didn't want to miss one minute of my birthday by staying in bed. The tradition continued, colorful decorations and my mom smiling brightly greeting me.

While I ate breakfast, Jimmy came downstairs, wished me a happy birthday and gave me two presents. First, he told me that last night, he texted Anthony and ask him about working for my mom. Anthony said yes. I called it a present because I figured Jimmy couldn't be too mad at Anthony if he asked him to be at our house every day to work. And that also meant I was going to get to see Anthony a lot more, granted behind a lawn mower or covered with paint, but, hey, I'd take it!

The second present was four tickets for *Singing in the Rain* that was playing at the Goodspeed Opera House in East Haddam, not too far from my house. The show was in three weeks. I hugged him and thanked him for his thoughtful gift. He knew how much I loved theater. I immediately told him I wanted him to come with us. And Anthony's sister, Chelsea.

A birthday lunch followed with my friends Kelly and Daniela at the Rainforest Café. My dad had a family party planned for that weekend.

Promptly at six, o'clock, wearing a white sundress with yellow flowers and a yellow bow around the waist, I opened the door and my mouth dropped. Anthony was dressed in a suit and I almost flipped. He was so handsome. When I was at his house a few weeks ago, I looked at the many pictures scattered on tables around the living room and hanging on the walls that showed the Dellaripa family dressed up for some special occasion, but to see Anthony all decked out in person was a whole other scene. He carried a little gift bag. He told me I looked pretty and wished me a happy birthday as he handed me the bag. I sat down on the couch, opened it and tears sprung from my eyes. The bag was filled with Sour Patch Kids, only the red and green ones.

"I bought two bags and picked out all the red and the green ones to make you a customized bag."

Totally impressed would be an understatement. I was thunderstruck that he put so much thought into a present for me. I couldn't stop hugging and thanking him. My mother came into the room, said hello to Anthony, and smiled. She kissed me good-bye and told us both to have fun. I wondered whether Anthony felt as weird as I did that every other time he came over, it was to hang with Jimmy, not take Jimmy's kid sister out on a date.

Laura's Journal

> When Anthony showed up to take Felicia to dinner for her birthday, he looked so cute with his button-down shirt and pants that were neither baggy nor jeans! Felicia came down the stairs wearing the cutest summer dress–white with yellow flowers–and Anthony blurted out, "You look so pretty!" that seemed to catch them both by surprise.
>
> Last week at her graduation, I kept saying to her father, "She wasn't supposed to be here." Every accomplishment, every struggle, every breath was an added amazement to the gift that is Felicia. Her whole life I tried to stay positive, knowing there is a fine line between optimism and denial, all the while praying she would know the safety of a good and kind love but at the same time wondering who would be strong enough for the unknown. When I saw Felicia's eyes light up as soon as she saw Anthony, I hoped and prayed he might be the one to have that strength for Felicia. I am so grateful that she now knows what being with a gentleman is like and pray he will continue to have the strength for her.

We headed north away from the shore. It was a warm night and we had the windows down. The balmy breeze felt so inviting as we drove. I had no idea where he was taking me and expected him to turn off at each exit off Route 9. Thirty minutes later he got off the highway, weaved his way through the streets of downtown Hartford, and pulled up in front of Max Downtown, one of the most upscale restaurants in the city.

We entered the restaurant, and, immediately, the hostess wished me a happy birthday and referred to me by name. I didn't think anything of it, assuming when Anthony made the reservation, he probably mentioned it was my birthday. But as we followed the hostess to our table, waiters passing us said, "Happy Birthday, Felicia." I turned to Anthony, who simply shrugged. But I didn't believe that he didn't have anything to do with it. The mystery was later solved when Anthony found out the next day his mother was the conspirator. She had offered to make the reservation for him and arranged with the manager for all staff members to wish me a happy birthday.

As the waiter cleared the table after dinner, Anthony excused himself to use the men's room. I looked around the room and felt like Cinderella. Cinderella Pascarella. What a perfect name!

Anthony returned and asked me if I wanted dessert. I shrugged. He said he wasn't the surprise-me-with-a-cake-type person who involved a group of waiters surrounding me and singing "Happy Birthday" as I blew out the candle while the rest of the patrons looked on. He didn't want to embarrass me in case that wasn't my thing either. He also said he didn't know what I liked. For the few times we had been together before and after our first date, I had never eaten anything except ice cream. He said we could stop somewhere on the way home if I wanted ice cream.

Just as he finished his little explanation, the waiter approached us with a tray full of desserts. I figured he was going to point to each dessert, describe it, and ask if we'd be interested in any of them. I expected Anthony to tell him we didn't want dessert. But instead of starting any descriptions, the waiter put the entire tray down.

"*Bon appetit, Mademoiselle* Felicia." And he walked away.

Confused, I turned to Anthony, who smiled sheepishly and confessed he didn't really need to go to the men's room. Because he didn't know what I liked for dessert, he ordered everything on the menu.

Red and green Sour Patch Kids and every dessert in the restaurant. Could he get any more romantic?

We took a taste of everything on the tray, chocolate chip ice cream cake with chocolate and caramel sauce and candied macadamia nuts, apple tart with caramel ice cream, chocolate mousse tower with raspberry coulis sauce, pistachio crème brûlée made with pistachio crunch, chocolate peanut butter molten cake with white chocolate crisp and ganache, a small bowl filled with small scoops of their ice cream and sorbet flavors of the day, and Max's signature cheesecake. We ate until we both felt like we were going to burst, and Anthony asked the waiter to wrap up the rest.

On the way out, I thanked all the waitstaff and said they helped make my birthday celebration with my friend so much more fun.

As this perfect night wound down and Anthony drove us back to the shore, I couldn't stop thanking him for my perfect evening.

"You know how you thanked the waiters?" Anthony asked.

"Yes?" I was confused why he was asking this question.

"Well, you, ah, said, it made the evening more fun with your *friend*."

"And?"

"And so you can call me your *boy*friend."

"Really?" I definitely felt like Cinderella now.

"And can I ask how my *girl*friend has liked her birthday so far?"

"Well, ah, *Boy*friend, you may. It couldn't be more Cinderella."

We stopped at a light and he leaned over and kissed me.

"You realize you accomplished something else today by turning eighteen other than being able to vote."

"I did?"

Other than my gluttonous attack on the array of the most decadent desserts, I couldn't figure out what he was talking about.

"You changed the statistics of cystic fibrosis survivors."

We pulled up to my house, and Anthony insisted he walk me in. Now that I knew Anthony liked to surprise me, I became suspicious. I tried to figure out why he insisted on walking me in and not just to the door. Would I be greeted by a room full of friends who'd jump out from behind my couch and shout, "Surprise"?

We entered the house and all was quiet except for the sound of the television coming from the den, where we found my mother on the couch and no one jumping out from behind it. She casually looked up, smiled, asked us if we had a good time. Anthony handed her the bag of desserts. Said to enjoy them, then asked her permission to go up to my room. Some lame excuse–or what I considered lame as I figured the surprise shouters were hiding there–about another gift he wanted to give me. I never saw the secret wink between Anthony and my mother.

We walked upstairs. When I opened the door to my bedroom, I let out a shout of surprise before the tears came gushing down. My bed was completely covered with tiny red roses. I didn't have to count the roses to know there were sixty-five of them.

Chapter Eight

The day before I was supposed to leave for the New Hampshire trip with Kelly, I had a doctor's appointment. For this one, Kelly offered to go with my mom and me. My dad would meet us there.

I was getting ready to head to the appointment when I heard the car door slam and knew it was Anthony reporting for his first day of work. I snuck a look out the window. He looked so cute wearing a paint-stained T-shirt. Impulse told me to run outside and hug him, but I knew that might not be the coolest thing to do his first day. Maybe another time. But nothing in my heart told me I couldn't stare at my boyfriend. I saw Jimmy approach him and say something about the other kid wouldn't be starting until the next week. I saw Anthony nod, then hold out his hand to shake Jimmy's. What was that all about?

Then I heard Anthony say, "You know, man, I'm sorry."

"I don't care about the whole never-date-a-sibling thing," Jimmy answered. "That was high school stuff. I just wish I wasn't the last to know."

"I should have told you about Felicia right away."

"It's OK. She's my sister. I worry about her."

They both nodded and then headed into the shed. I couldn't see or hear them anymore.

On the drive to the doctor's appointment, Kelly and I sat in the backseat, and she told me her boyfriend was coming up to the cottage for the weekend and Anthony was invited also. That sounded fun so I texted him and he said yes!

Before I did the usual PFT test to measure my lung capacity, Dr. P announced she had something to say.

"This is our first appointment since passing the estimated two-year mark for Felicia's survival without a lung transplant. I'm most pleased as I'm sure all of you are."

My mother piped up. "One month, three weeks, six days. And her graduation was one month, two weeks, three days past the date."

The silence in the room was intense as my mother wiped her tearing eyes.

"Um . . . yes, and that was what I also wanted to say." Dr. P turned to me directly. "Congratulations. I know what these last four years have been like with your health and I know how much you love school. To see you be so dedicated to your studies and do your homework even while in the hospital was admirable."

I nodded my thanks. I was still reeling from both Dr. P's and my mother's comments. I had actually forgotten about that two-year mark until just now. It's not as though I kept a calendar, crossing off each day to count how long I had to live if I didn't have the transplant. Evidently, others had kept track.

"But, Felicia, I also don't want you to disillusion yourself. Your lungs are working at less capacity than two years ago, so we are not going in the right direction. As you well know, I can no more force you to put your name on the transplant list now than before."

She ended with a smile and handed me the tube to start my PFT test. She looked at the result, raised her eyebrows, and asked me do it a second time. Again, I blew into the tube, but the results were no better than the first. My PFT numbers were low. I didn't need her to say anything. Having lived with CF for eighteen years, I didn't need my doctor to tell me the next step. I needed to have a bronch. I knew I was due for one, but these numbers mandated one a lot sooner. I spoke up before she did.

"But Kelly and I are going to New Hampshire tomorrow." I pointed to Kelly as though she were Exhibit A in a courtroom, like her being there would validate changing my doctor's mind. I also kept my eyes focused on her, so I wouldn't have to see the disapproving stare of my mom, as she probably surmised I was about to ask the so-called unthinkable. *Can it wait a few days?* That she was very used to with me.

"When are you leaving?" Dr. P asked.

"Tomorrow. And my boyfriend is coming up on Saturday for a night." (My absent Exhibit B.)

"And when are you coming back?"

Now I heard my mother squirm. I knew she was definitely getting upset because I bet she'd already assumed there was no way my doctor would ever let me go. I was half-waiting for Dr. P to do the "if only I did my meds" lecture, but bronchs were becoming pretty routine for everyone with CF, and even though doing meds may have some effect on the frequency of bronchs, it was not necessarily an equation. People who religiously follow their CF protocol still need bronchs periodically, because meds can only do so much to keep the lungs mucus-free. The others just may not need bronchs as often as an eighteen-year-old rebel with CF. What wasn't the same on both sides of the equation was doing meds religiously and being guaranteed never to need a lung transplant.

"In a week. Next Wednesday."

Dr. P was silent, stared at my file, looked up at me.

"Come home Sunday. Be at the hospital at six Monday morning."

She turned to Kelly and said with a sweet yet emphatic tone, "You make sure she spends at least two hours a day–not all at once, of course–hiking, swimming, anything to keep those lungs moving."

"Cross my heart and lungs," Kelly giggled.

"Now, go pack, and have seven days of fun in four."

I clapped for joy. Kelly clapped for joy. My father was stoic. My mom was surprised and frustrated. I had already started to text Anthony.

So Felicia was going into the hospital. Another first in our new relationship with my girlfriend. But I knew this was always a possibility. As long as Felicia smiled, I knew I'd be OK. Whatever our conversations, all she had to do was flash me one of those bright smiles, and if I was down about something, I immediately perked up. Felicia had already filled me in on what a bronch was like and what to expect, so I was prepared for this hospitalization. As prepared as you can be in life when you're twenty and dating a girl with CF.

True to her word, Kelly made sure I stayed active. For three days, we hiked, canoed, and took long walks along the lake. We did girly-girl things: sat on the dock painting our toenails, waving our toes in the air under the warm sun to dry them. At night, we watched reruns of the *Gilmore Girls*–something we knew neither of the guys would ever watch.

I knew I missed being with Anthony but didn't realize just

how much until Saturday morning when I saw his car pull into the driveway. How would I ever survive when he went back to college at the end of the summer? But that wasn't for weeks and today was today.

First on the agenda for the four of us was a trip into town to walk around. Swinging our hands as we strolled through the quaint streets, Anthony and I wandered into a woodcarving place where we observed artists transform a solid block of wood into ducks, baskets, and Christmas ornaments. We passed a Harley-Davidson store and decided to go in because we thought it'd be fun to look at the different kinds of bikes, helmets and other accessories. After eating hot dogs, fries and ice cream cones, we drove back to the cottage and sprawled on the dock as we digested lunch before jumping into the water.

After a few hours, Anthony and I decided to take the rowboat out. Kelly and her boyfriend wanted to stay on the dock and swim.

It was late in the afternoon and the water was so calm I could lean over the side and see my reflection. With very few people on the lake, it was so peaceful. No one around to ask us questions, to judge us. *How could she date someone if she knows she has a serious disease? How can he date her and not worry every minute she will die?*

"Remember when I asked you about how you knew you had CF?"

"I remember everything you ask me."

Anthony faltered for a minute as though he wasn't expecting an answer anywhere close to that one.

"How old were you when you realized what you had?"

The short answer would have been to simply say eight years old, and stop at that, but I felt Anthony deserved to hear more. If he was starting to open up and ask more questions, I wanted him to understand me. I didn't want unanswered questions to be a barrier to our relationship. It was also at that moment I realized that hearing about me meant to share my lung transplant story. That was definitely going to happen before we rowed back to shore.

One question led to another. I felt a mix of relief as he began to understand the layers beneath the surface of my CF, but also fears that at any one point a piece of information might drive him away.

"I was eight years old," I answered and quickly recounted the story about how I was in third grade and had to leave school, be in a hospital for the first time, and miss my trip to visit my grandparents.

"So that day, even though I was only eight, I finally understood I had a serious disease."

Anthony hesitated, them sputtered, "Like you could . . . ah . . . ."

I let go of the oar and touched his hand.

"Anthony, you can say the word *die*. It's not like I don't know it. And the answer is no. Not until seventh grade."

I picked up the oar and started to row again.

"There was this new kid at my school and I had a huge crush on him, so on the bus on the way home from school, I made sure I sat next to him. We were talking about something funny that happened in geography that day when I started to cough. A three or a four. I pulled out my inhaler and the coughing finally stopped. He looked scared and I explained I had CF and it made me cough a lot. Anyhow, by this time in my life, word of mouth overpowered my desire to keep CF to myself and everyone in school knew about it. He asked me whether I could die from it. I kind of freaked. That's the first time I ever heard the word *die* in terms of CF. I just shrugged. The second I got home, I stormed into the house and asked my mom.

"My mother sat me down on the couch, put her arm around me and said, 'Felicia, honey, yes, you can die, but everyone dies. Your heart has a certain amount of beats and one day, runs out of them.' She always talked so gently to me. She told me that I had nothing to worry about.

"A few months later, my mother and I were watching that Adam Sandler film, *Little Nicky*, and it was about dying. I turned to her and asked, 'If I die when I am sixteen, will I always be sixteen in heaven?'"

I always thought it was kind of spooky–and ironic–that I happened to pick the number sixteen because of the whole transplant thing. I knew this was the moment I had to bring up this big part of my life. I felt our relationship had reached a level that not telling him about the transplant would be irresponsible. He had to know that my health would always be precarious because of CF. That, even though I had passed the two-year marker, my condition was still tenuous. This last comment could be my transition into the lung transplant.

"I know that was a long answer to a simple question. I'm sorry."

"Hey, don't be," Anthony, answered. "These must be hard things to talk about."

This was my moment. *You have no idea how hard. You see, CF people can need lung transplants. No. Ironically, I picked sixteen, because a few years later, when I really was sixteen, I found out . . . . No. Anthony, there is something really important I need you to know. A few years ago, I–*

"I have a pretty tough story. A life-changing moment, not to sound dramatic," Anthony blurted out.

"Oh?" I looked at his face scrunched up in a weird expression, and I cocked my head–sign language to go ahead and tell me.

"Sometimes, my mother has to travel for her job. A few years ago, she had been scheduled to drive to Boston for a meeting and then fly to California for another meeting. So she finished her Boston meeting on a Monday night and the next morning, drove to the airport to fly to California. But before she reached the airport, her secretary called to tell her that the California meeting was postponed and my mom was to drive back to Connecticut. She called my dad but only got his voice mail, so she left him a message and started driving home. She was planning to surprise Andrew, Chelsea and me and be at home when we got back from school. Problem was . . . ah . . . she didn't have the radio on and hadn't heard back from my dad. I was at school when all chaos . . . ."

Anthony stopped, sucked in a breath. I started to ask if he was OK when he continued.

"She had been booked on one of the planes . . . to LA . . . the World Trade Center . . . September 11, 2001."

He just completely stopped rowing, as I understood what he was telling me. If his mother's meeting hadn't been canceled, she would have boarded that plane. *And* he knew about the attack before he knew his mother was OK.

Carefully, I leaned over, trying not to rock the boat too much, and hugged him. Although we'd only been dating a few weeks, I felt our relationship had deepened into another level. I was always the one with the intense stories. Aside from admitting a fear of roller coasters, Anthony had yet to open up to me about much.

How do I even tell him my news after that? He seemed so relieved to tell me his story, almost cathartic. Yet he also seemed emotionally spent and we were up here to have fun on a trip already cut short. But what if . . . ?

"Anthony, there's one more thing you need to know."

I never expected Felicia to tell me such an intense story. Refusing a lung transplant! But I'm not in her shoes, so who am I to say what I would do? And she told me this story two months after some time frame about dying. I can't imagine what it's like for her to get up every morning with this disease hanging over her head. Something that never goes away. My mom's experience made me see the possibilities that death can be close to home. Made me appreciate life more. Since then, I don't take being with anybody for granted because death can strike at any moment.

Now this? But where do I fit in? Just keep dating her and

having fun? I think I already know my answer to that. She did seem to be a miracle child. Refused a lung transplant over two years ago. Did have a stent put in that was temporary for a few weeks and that was almost two years ago.

She has such a spirit of life; she gives me a spirit. I'll take that.

For the rest of the day, we couldn't stop hugging and kissing and holding hands, or just staring at each other to make sure we were both real to one another. We had truly opened our souls as we rowed on the lake.

That night we swung on a glider on the porch. Kelly and her boyfriend chose the Adirondack chairs. Suddenly, Kelly said we should make S'mores and hopped up to go in the house. I offered to help but she said that I should stay with Anthony, and she grabbed her boyfriend's hand.

As soon as they were out of sight, Anthony leaned over and kissed me and I started to cough. This CF nemesis of coughing while kissing had been on my I-hate-CF list ever since I was old enough to have my first kiss. Luckily, I didn't have to cough the first time ever a boy kissed me, so at least I have a good memory of that first in my life. But I wasn't so lucky other times boys kissed me, and I was always nervous when kissing. I pulled away from Anthony and, this time, I wasn't nervous! I finished coughing and I laughed. Anthony laughed and he kissed me again and life went on.

And then all too soon, it was Sunday afternoon, and we needed to get on the road back to Connecticut. I suggested that Anthony and I go home and Kelly and her boyfriend could stay. But they said no and we all went back home. Short as my trip was, at least I got to go and still had fun with Anthony. On the way home, I realized I never got nervous that anything would happen to me in those few days. I figured no doctor would let me out of her sight if I were really that sick and tried not to think about the fact that as soon as I got home, I needed to go into the hospital. But I had to. And I did.

Chapter Nine

Just like the other times I have been hospitalized for a bronch, I was an in-patient for four days, mostly to receive the postbronch IV antibiotics. Dr. P always starts them with intensity in the hospital. After four days, I am free to go home to complete the course of antibiotics with my pic line.

Anthony had stayed at my house the night before so he could help take my mother and me to the hospital early the next morning. Someone always came with us, whether one of my girlfriends or guy friends. And my dad, as always, drove up from his house to meet us there. He lived west of Yale Hospital and we lived east of it.

My mother always liked that I had a friend come along for extra support. She never let a friend come in the recovery room, though–a place where a lot of kids cried or screamed. It was hard enough for me, once I woke up. I remember one particularly tough time when I heard a little girl scream that she couldn't feel her legs. Broke my heart. And I wasn't the prettiest sight to see–vomiting up blood, typical of a postbronch.

Once in my own room, no friends were allowed to see me

until my mother cleared it. The vomiting would continue for a few hours, but with less intensity as time passed, so once I got over the initial bout, my mother would then allow my friends to come in the room to see me.

Having my dad sleep overnight with me at the hospital brought many special moments beyond the visitation agreements between my mother and him. It's not that we ever went into deep philosophical discussions like my mom and I do. Our relationship was based solely on special times together. And it's not that he didn't impact my life. I know he felt awful and confused by my decision as everyone else did. He just said what he had to say about that in a few words–and a few words can say a lot–and then used looks and glances that spoke volumes. As he always says to me, "I'm your dad, and I will always give you the look."

My dad would watch *Gilmore Girls* episodes with me because he knew how much I liked them. He'd sit by my bed in a large family chair that converted to a bed, and with each episode, I'd have to fill him in on what was happening on the show because, he, like Anthony, didn't usually watch it.

One of my hospital visits included more than a bronch. I had been having a lot of sore throats and sinus problems, so Dr. P operated on my sinuses and took out my tonsils in addition to doing a bronch. That night I had a lot of bleeding and instead of calling the nurses, each time I needed the gauze changed, my dad stayed up with me all night wiping my nose and changing gauze.

Anthony stayed with me until I was wheeled into the operating room; then he paced the waiting room until Dr. P finished the bronch and delivered news that all was OK. (My mother told me this later. "Up and down, up and down.") Once out of the procedure and once he got my mother's all-clear signal, he came in to see me.

When Anthony walked in the room, if my looks or all the tubes in me shocked him, he didn't show it or say anything.

True to his typical ways, he smiled, sat down, and stroked my hand.

Tuesday morning, Anthony arrived at the hospital at ten, armed with games, magazines, and DVDs. My mother, Jimmy, Kelly, Nick, and other friends revolved in and out of the room at various times, and, later, my father came for the night. I was never left alone. Someone was always with me.

When Anthony left at the end of the day, I thanked him over and over for staying with me. As much as I relished the day with him by my side, I told him that he didn't have to come back the next morning, and I'd be home in three days. He nodded knowingly. The next morning, he arrived at ten, armed with more games, magazines, and DVDs. Although elated to see him, I told him again he didn't have to visit me, and he again nodded. For the next two days until I was discharged, he showed up armed with different games, magazines, and movies. He even sat through an episode of the *Gilmore Girls*–and paid attention. What a guy!

Being the boyfriend requires me to respect Felicia and the decisions she makes throughout life because it is her life. However, I must do what is right and tell her how I feel, because all relationships require fairness and respect. So while she recuperated from the latest bronch, I shared my concerns about her decision not to have the lung transplant but balanced that by honoring her decision about her life. Almost as tough to say that kind of stuff as it was to see her in the hospital bed with tubes coming out of her. I was scared before going to the hospital, but once I saw her after she woke up, I was cool with it all. Besides, being her boyfriend means that I will be there for her. I made a commitment.

Early in the afternoon of the fourth day at the hospital, Anthony drove my mother and me home from the hospital. Later, Kelly stopped by. In spite of being tired, I wanted to go outside and get some fresh air, so Kelly, Anthony, and I went out for pizza and came back to watch a DVD. The day seemed endless, and it wasn't even five o'clock!

As usual, once at home from the hospital, I had a new schedule of medicines. For three weeks I had to have IV antibiotics in my pic line. I needed four doses a day of one of the antibiotics: six a.m., noon, six p.m., and midnight; then I had another antibiotic I needed once a day right after my noon dose of the first antibiotic. Finish the noon dose; flush the pic line with a saline solution and insert the one p.m. medicine. I also had to do chest percussions three or four times a day and add two rounds of the breathing machine. These were all extra precautions to make sure the lungs were clear after the bronch. Even if I were in a rebellion stage, I always did my postbronch schedule religiously. I didn't want to end up back in the hospital with complications and more antibiotics.

At five-thirty, my mother came into the kitchen. Our den and kitchen are actually one open room. She asked how I was feeling. I looked up to answer but also noticed Anthony staring at my mother as she opened the refrigerator to take out the bottle of medicine to warm it up. He didn't say anything and turned back to watch the movie. But when she returned to the kitchen twenty minutes later, again his attention was on my mother and not the television. He watched her as she washed her hands thoroughly, picked up the warmed bottle of medicine, and headed toward the couch. Kelly moved away so my mother could sit down next to me. Anthony continued to watch intensely while she flushed the pic line with a saline solution, cleaned the end of the pic, cleaned the top of the bottle, and connected the bottle to the pic line. If my mother moved in a way to block his view of my pic line, he craned his neck.

What was he doing? All I could think of was that he was freaking. If seeing me in the hospital gown and vomiting didn't get to him, maybe this did. Having compassion for me because I have CF, saying he was sorry for me when I told him stories of my life, and trying to imagine what my life was like was only one side of the fence. Actually witnessing my life was way on the other side. Sure he got a glimpse of it in the hospital and seemed OK with it, but others were taking care of me then. Every time a doctor or nurse came in to do any procedure, visitors were asked to leave the room. As my mother did the last step of pushing the bottle onto the needle, Anthony raised his eyebrows and watched even more intensely. I wondered whether he was thinking, *What if I have to do this for her?* I figured he'd bail; say he got himself involved in more than he had realized. I stopped eyeing him because I was afraid to see his expression.

By six o'clock, the bottle was attached with the antibiotics entering my body. It would take an hour to complete the dose. My mother said she'd be back in an hour and left the room. Anthony never said a word and concentrated on the television. I'd say he didn't hug me or rub my arm or kiss my hair while I had the bottle in me, but Kelly had plunked herself back down on the couch between us to help decorate little armbands to cover the pic line, or, as I nicknamed them, "stare blockers."

My mother came back at seven to take out the bottle. (It's crucial to take it out once the bottle is empty because blood can back up into my lungs if the bottle has nothing in it.) I watched Anthony out of the corner of my eye. Again, he eyed my mother intently. He even followed her into the kitchen, saying he was getting a Coke. Why? To explain to her that he was breaking up with me so she could be ready to comfort me? That would be so typical of his thoughtfulness. But at this point, I was beginning to panic.

Did I bite off more than I could handle in dating Felicia? Can I do this? Can I take care of Felicia the way she is depending on me to do? Am I responsible enough? This is way more than I ever imagined that first night I texted her. Can I measure up to what she needs? I'm being selfish. No, I'm not. I'm not questioning this for selfish reasons. What if I can't take care of Felicia the way she needs me to? I guess you don't know what you're in for until you take the ride. I know by choosing to date Felicia, I got more than I bargained for. A lot more. But then again, I'd have to have been crazy not to ask her out. I just didn't know just how much being her boyfriend entailed.

Soon after Kelly went home, my mother came in to tell me that she was going up to bed and that she would get up later to do my midnight treatment. Although I could do the IV meds myself, my mother always got up to do the midnight and six a.m. treatments so I could get more sleep. A bronch treatment took a lot out of me. She thanked Anthony for all his help, bringing me home from the hospital and taking care of me. It was comforting that my mother liked Anthony so much.

I asked Anthony if he wanted to get going and he seemed reluctant to leave, so we put on another movie. I was so tired I kept drifting in and out of sleep until I couldn't follow the plot anymore, and the next thing I knew, I woke up on the couch with the morning sun streaming in. Confused, I looked around, and there was Anthony, fast asleep at the other end of the couch. I looked at the clock. It was eight in the morning. Obviously, my mother must have not woken him up when she came in to do my midnight and six a.m. treatments.

I lay on the couch thinking how happy I was that he was there, yet nervous because I knew that before he fell asleep, he must have made a decision to break it off with me. As soon as he woke up, he'd tell me. I looked at his sneakers that he had kicked off earlier in the evening and envisioned him jumping into them and running as far away as he could as fast as he could. And, really, could I blame him?

I thought about a conversation I had with my dad two nights before in the hospital. He remarked that he had always liked Anthony. That he is a hard worker. It takes a special guy to take care of me. That anyone could be good with someone when life is smooth, but when the road gets rough, will that person still be there for the person? And he was certain Anthony was that kind of guy. My dad wondered whether at that age, he would have been able–the way Anthony seemed to be doing with me–to take care of a girl who was sick. He guessed he would, and I told him I knew he would. I loved my dad so much. I felt so confident that my dad was right about Anthony. He drove us to the hospital and he came and visited me every day. But watching Anthony watch my mother last night took away that confidence.

My mother walked in and smiled. She bent down, gave me a kiss on my forehead, and whispered, "How are you?"

"Fine. Thanks for doing the treatments," I whispered.

"Don't thank me. Thank Anthony. He's the one who got up and did the midnight *and* the six a.m."

I gasped and my mother nodded.

"He sent you away?"

"No, Felicia. I was in the kitchen around nine having a glass of water. He walked over to me, said you had fallen asleep, and step-by-step told me how to do the antibiotics. He didn't miss one step. He said I didn't need to get up at midnight or six a.m. That he'd take care of it."

She winked and left the room, leaving me completely dumbfounded. I couldn't take my eyes off him. He looked so cute sleeping so soundly in his jeans and sweatshirt. How sweet of him. No, more than sweet. How generous. How strong. And here I was convinced he was freaking. I took out a magazine and quietly read while Anthony slept. But I found myself sitting with the same page on my lap, as I couldn't stop looking at him. I'd have to start my breathing machine and chest percussions in a little while, but for now all I wanted to do was stare at my boyfriend.

Jimmy entered and I pointed to Anthony asleep on the couch to stop him from talking. He nodded, headed into the kitchen, grabbed some juice out of the refrigerator, and held up the bottle miming did I want any. I shook my head. He gulped a glassful, mimed again pointing to the outside, and headed out the door. I returned to staring at Anthony.

For the next three weeks, Anthony stayed over and did my midnight and six a.m. meds. Anthony became a routine fixture in my house. He found the comfortable balance of making himself at home, yet still asking at times if it was okay if he got something out of the refrigerator despite the number of times my mother said he didn't have to ask. We all became so comfortable with each other that one day, when I asked my mother to do chest percussions on my back, she turned to Anthony and said, "Hey, you're a drummer. Why don't you drum on her back?"

Need I tell you Anthony's answer?

Most times I slept through the midnight and early morning doses of antibiotics. Occasionally, I'd wake up and instead of going back to sleep, I'd sit up with Anthony, and we'd talk for the hour until it was time to take the bottle out. I don't remember how we got on the topic of his "drinking it in" philosophy, but somehow we did. His dad taught him to get everything he could out of life. Like when going to the theater. He shouldn't just rush through the lobby, hand over the tickets to an usher, take a program and be shown to his seat. That he should take the time to look around at the lobby decor, the architecture, lighting, wall hangings, interesting sculpture, whatever surrounds him. And again, once inside the theater, look at the curtains, the balconies, sconces, anything to surround himself with the moment–to drink it in. I pointed out that that is one way to live in the moment, and Anthony said he never realized the connection. He just always thought his dad had taught him a cool thing. When I casually mentioned that I thought about opening a photography studio someday, he became very excited because he realized that if I were planning I must be thinking about a future! We were teaching each other!

Another night, I woke up and saw Anthony listening to my Ipod. He saw me stir and took off the Ipod.

"Hey, I didn't know you liked Nat King Cole. This is like the third one on this track."

"I have every single song of his on the Ipod. Which one is on?"

"*Unforgettable.*"

"My favorite."

I loved that we had already discovered so many things about each other and had fallen into a comfortable pattern of knowing each other's likes and dislikes. I loved how he paid attention to me–little things, like remembering I liked only red and green Sour Patch Kids. I knew he liked Monster, an energy drink, so I always tried to pick one up for him. But I equally loved that we were still discovering each other.

These weeks after my bronch brought us closer in ways I never could have imagined. Pretty intense to have a guy who after only three weeks of dating gets up at midnight, sets up my treatment, sits up for an hour while it does its thing, disconnects it, goes back to sleep, gets up at six a.m., and does it all over again–all while I sleep. No one other than my mom and dad has ever taken such care of me. I was very, very lucky to have Anthony in my life.

Laura's Journal

Shortly after Felicia started dating Anthony, she had another bronch and a short hospital stay to place the pic line and start IV treatments. Anthony was there the day of the bronch, the day after the bronch, the next day, and the next. Finally, I remarked to Felicia that I was impressed that he kept coming back; it was clear there was something unique and special happening between them.

We had all started a new dance. I had fewer steps while Felicia and Anthony learned a new rhythm that included meds and IVs and life outside of CF. Felicia and I are both benefiting from the strength of character, safety, and compassion of this young man!

Chapter Ten

The date on the tickets for *Singing in the Rain* that Jimmy had given me for my birthday fell during those three weeks on antibiotics. The four of us decided to have dinner out first. We chose La Vita Gustosa, the restaurant I had worked at, coincidentally around the corner from the Goodspeed.

Shortly before the bronch, I began to realize that working was really too much for me, and I decided to leave my job. I didn't make a big deal out of it. Just told my boss that my health had deteriorated somewhat, that I didn't feel good and that I didn't think it was wise to continue to work. He was very understanding.

Although I had only been at the restaurant for a short time, I had a sense of accomplishment–I learned that I could work. I had given working a try, and, in time, I hoped to have another job. Just not now. Like so many other aspects of my life, adjustments had to be made. I was used to it by now and, surprisingly, didn't have a what if? moment. I didn't ask myself, *What if I didn't have CF? Would I still be out there working?* Maybe, just maybe, I don't always have to dissect how CF affects my life. The key was not to worry about any future jobs. When the time is right, I know I want to work again. End of story.

It was fun to go back to see the people I had worked with, and they were all happy to see me. Some people might feel awkward going back to a place they once worked or not go at all. But I felt comfortable and welcomed by the warm reception I got. I excitedly introduced Anthony to everyone, and of course, I said, "Meet Anthony, my boyfriend."

After we ordered, I excused myself to go to the ladies' room. I came back just as our dinners arrived. I sat down, made sure the bottle of medicine was upright in my pocketbook, adjusted my armband that had slipped down and dug into my meal as my six p.m. course of antibiotics traveled through my pic line.

After dinner, Anthony and I walked hand in hand down the street to the theater with Chelsea and Jimmy on either side of us. Despite the wondrous evening so far, I had a what if? moment. *What if the tickets had been for when I was in the hospital?* I especially hated a what if? question after the fact because I wasn't in the hospital. I was on my way to a fun show with a guy I adored. I think I was equally bothered by even allowing a what if? question to seep into a perfect day. I didn't realize I had been stewing until Anthony, in a low voice, asked me if something was wrong.

"What if these tickets had been for when I was in the hospital?"

"Easy enough to exchange them." And he used a silly, goofy voice that he sometimes did to make me laugh, and it worked.

"Right. Easy. I know you're right. I just get frustrated about so many things. Like how it's important to be physically active to help my lungs and yet I have a time limit. I get winded before I'm ready to quit exercising. And that's just one thing on my list of things I hate about having CF."

"You have a rating list for those like your coughs?"
"No. I've always hated them equally."

The Goodspeed Opera House sits in an idyllic setting on the Connecticut River. The sunlight glistens on the river, and at night, the building's lights reflect on the darkened water. Goodspeed is a Victorian-style building with perfect acoustics. Built in the late 1800s, the first show opened in 1877. I loved the history of the opera house, how it became a militia base during World War I, then a general store and even a storage building for a state agency. It began to deteriorate and was targeted to be torn down, but a group of dedicated citizens in the mid-60s fought to restore it to a theater. Some shows have even started here before going on to Broadway. It is by far one of my favorite places to go, which is why my brother gave me the tickets. Just as I had taught Anthony to live in the moment, once inside, he showed me how to "drink it in" and absorb every detail like his father taught him.

I smiled, laughed, and clapped my way through the lively, boisterous singing and dancing. At intermission, we stepped out onto a terrace, with its wrought iron tables and chairs, and we watched the river flow. The daytime heat had disappeared and a balmy breeze had taken its place. Anthony and I leaned over the rail, our arms wrapped around one another, and watched the illuminated water flow. Then we walked back in for the second half of the show.

When Felicia had to excuse herself to start her antibiotics at dinner, I was so frustrated at how CF interrupts her life. Chelsea and Jimmy were talking away and all I could do was picture Felicia putting down the toilet seat, washing her hands, shaking the bottle, preparing to put in the needle, sitting on the top of the toilet, injecting it into the pic line, putting the armband back on.

After intermission, I found myself looking more at Felicia than at the stage. She had this cool pink shirt with a matching pink armband, and she was tapping her foot to Broadway Rhythm. *She totally blows my mind. Like, she had just been so frustrated about a* what if? *moment and maybe missing the show, and now here she was, bubbly and happy. It just amazes me how quickly she can bounce back from a bad mood and negative thoughts. She wasn't kidding when she said she lives in the moment. Me? I hope I, too, wouldn't wallow, but I doubt my mood could shift as quickly as Felicia's. Like when I worried that I haven't gotten my grades for the semester yet, or I agonized over whether I signed up for the best courses to take next semester or . . . .*

A few days after the show, a visiting nurse came to the house to remove my pic line and I was done with that–until the next bronch or infection, or who knows what happens to me. A week later was my checkup, and I brought a new friend. When I asked Anthony if he wanted to go with me, he readily agreed, which both comforted me and made me anxious. The comforted feeling was obvious, but being nervous confused me. It was like being afraid to get on a step stool after having climbed Mt. Everest. He had already seen me vomit blood in the hospital, had wiped sweat off my forehead, and spent three weeks disturbing his sleep to do my meds. Yet I still thought sitting in Dr. P's office would be too much. I worried about nothing. Dr. P gave Anthony a "lecture" that combined accolades for his dedication to me and a directive that he get on my case to continue my meds, breathing machine and chest percussions. Other than telling Kelly to make sure I exercised in New Hampshire, Dr. P had never given any directives. My mother sat quietly.

On the way home from the appointment, Anthony and I were both kind of quiet. When he pulled into my driveway, I simply said, "If this gets too tough for you, I'll understand."

He shook his head, leaned over, gave me a long kiss and said he had to get to work. He hopped out of the car and headed toward the shed that housed the lawn mower, turned back, and winked at me. How did he know I would be standing there staring at him and smiling?

The summer days fell into a pattern. Anthony painted or worked on the lawn, and I continued to recreate my world through the lens of my camera. On weekends, we took long walks on the beach or swam. At night, we stared at the stars or we swayed to the music at Bill's. What we didn't do was spend any more time taking me to hospitals or bronchs, and I was better about my meds. Not perfect. But better. Anthony was the loving taskmaster, never allowing a day to go by without asking whether I'd done them. I never lied and he never chastised me when I said I hadn't, but I knew I could add him to the list of disappointed people for not doing them.

We began to go out with other couples, either friends we already knew together or some of his I hadn't yet met and vice versa. Just as I had wondered how much Jimmy had told Anthony about me when we first dated, I was curious how much his friends knew about me. Eventually, I asked Anthony after he introduced me to new friends whether he told them about my CF. Sometimes he had, and other times, he never said anything. I'm not even sure why I cared, other than that I didn't want the stares or pitying looks when I met new people. Actually, one of the most common statements I get when people find out I have CF is, "You don't look sick." I laugh and say, "I know."

That summer together, we also never got to Six Flags or any amusement park or any place that had a roller coaster ride.

Seems every time I convinced Anthony to go, he hesitated but always finally gave in to me. Yet something always messed up the plans, whether a social conflict or rain. I think Anthony was secretly relieved. At least I had gone there several times with Kelly during our spring vacation, and that roller coaster fix would have to sustain me for the summer. Next summer? Now that was another story.

One night in early August, I was at Anthony's house. It was still 80 degrees and very humid at nine o'clock at night– the clothes-stick-to-your-skin kind of humidity–so we didn't even want to sit outside. While watching a DVD instead, my cell phone rang that I had a text. It was from the boyfriend I had broken up with just before Anthony came along. He was having family problems and asked my advice. I held up the cell phone to show Anthony the caller ID and put up my finger to indicate that I'd only be a minute. Then I texted back an answer. But that minute lasted longer than I had intended. I'd answer a question; gave him my best advice that led to another text and another and another. This pattern continued for almost half an hour. I kept inching myself away from Anthony to be quieter. I wanted to put an end to these texts and began to shorten my answers, but like a boomerang, I'd get another text and toss out another response, hoping it'd be the last one.

A few times, I heard Anthony sigh and reposition himself on the couch. Finally, he stopped the DVD, and told me how rude I was, sitting with him, yet texting away with someone else. He said that even though I was being quiet, my attention wasn't on him and I should have just sent back a message that I couldn't "talk" right now. He said he's all for helping out other people and appreciated that I was kind, but I was still being impolite. That if I felt it was that crucial to help the guy, I should have excused myself and gone home to do so.

Wow! This was a new side of Anthony. He didn't yell, wasn't insulting, just calmly announced all this in a matter-of-fact voice.

"Besides, isn't he the same guy you told me didn't even visit when you were in the hospital last year? Let him find someone else to give him therapy."

I put my cell away, sat quietly and, eventually, the gap between us on the couch lessened. I ended up cuddled under his arm after an "I'm sorry" and got a gentle kiss on my head in return.

This was a major step in our relationship. Although not an all-out fight, it was the first time we were annoyed with each other: Anthony with me for what he considered rudeness and me for thinking Anthony wasn't understanding that although I broke up with this guy months ago, he needed me.

So we each found the other wasn't perfect, had our first annoyance, and got over it.

Then there was the rabbit.

On the way home from a movie or the beach, I can't remember exactly when, Anthony blurted out, "Let's go get a rabbit."

"Now?"

"You said you wanted one."

"Ten minutes ago. I swear, Anthony Dellaripa, you talk about me being spontaneous!"

"You're a good teacher. Besides, I think it's a good idea. Like we should see if we could share a big responsibility."

"What would we name it? I mean he or she?" I was so flabbergasted.

"I'm not *that* spontaneous. You pick a name."

We named her Rory. She was soft, adorable, had gray eyes, white paws and, unfortunately, didn't last a very long time at my house. The first afternoon I wheezed, Rory looked at me with her big eyes as though to ask, "What's wrong, Felicia?" As soon as I put Rory in the cage in my den and left the room, I stopped wheezing. With only one puff of my inhaler, I was fine. By that weekend, if I even walked to the edge of the room and tried to look at her, the wheezing started again.

I hated to tell Anthony that rabbit fur affected my lungs, but if we were going to have an honest relationship, I needed to let him know I couldn't keep the rabbit. In truth, I had suspected the rabbit fur was going to be a problem. Finally, I got the courage to tell him. Nothing super magnanimous on my part. The next time he came over and wanted to pat the rabbit, I had to fess up. He took it in true Anthony style. Immediately, he said how sorry he was.

Rory now lives happily ever after in the Dellaripa household in Anthony's bedroom.

A week after Rory took up her new residence, Anthony had an appointment to have his wisdom teeth out. Let's just say he wasn't exactly the best patient, something he owns up to. He admits he could have been a little less whiny, less needy and less complaint-ridden. This interesting reversal of patient and caretaker also deepened our relationship as I hovered like a mother hen. *Can I get you this? Can I do this? Make you that?* He said part of his poor patient behavior was his strong aversion to being taken care of, despite his complaining.

I brought him magazines, DVDs, and games; boiled water and made tea, fluffed his pillows, and soothed him.

I loved being a caretaker.

Chapter Eleven

As the sun began to set earlier each day, my live-in-the-moment philosophy was put to a test. I had one eye on having fun and the other on the dwindling days of summer, which would inevitably mean it was time for Anthony to leave for college. We hadn't been apart for a single day since my trip to New Hampshire.

While every second with Anthony was special, not to sound trite, some moments stuck out more than others, two in particular during those last weeks before summer disappeared.

One day, I needed to meet Anthony at the beach because of my schedule. I found him near the ocean's edge. He was talking animatedly with an older man and woman I didn't recognize and assumed to be some friends of his parents. Anthony flung his arm around my shoulder and introduced me as his girlfriend. *Girlfriend.* Even after dating for two months, hearing Anthony say that word still gave me butterflies. The couple smiled, thanked Anthony for all his advice, and walked on.

I looked at Anthony confused.

"What was that about?"

"Oh, they're down from Maine. I was just telling them the great places to go here and some good restaurants."

I grinned at Anthony.

"What's that smirk for?"

"Nothing."

"That isn't a nothing smirk."

"You're happy to have tourists here. Remember how you hated them invading your town in summer?"

Anthony laughed, "Yeah, yeah, yeah."

The other significant event happened during a stargazing night, only a few days before Anthony had to leave for school.

"What did you think about the night you asked me out?" I suddenly blurted out, but not until I found Orion's Belt. I never talked until I found the stars I knew.

"Besides I was glad your name started with an F?"

"Oh, I forgot about that whole first name in address book thing. Anything else?"

"I remember when we finally texted good-bye. Like, what was it, three in the morning? I was happy you'd go out with me, and I started remembering that time in high school. I think it was my junior year when I came over to your house to hang with Jimmy and you walked into the den. How you didn't look so good and had a huge bruise on one arm and some kind of tubing sticking out of it. I mean, I knew what you had, but I never saw you like that. I didn't know that much about the disease except from what I heard people say. Like you are born with it and don't usually live a long life. Funny, I had no idea the tubing was called a pic line. Things are way different now."

He leaned over and kissed me.

"Good different," he assured me. "What did you think about?"

"That your name started with an A."

"Yeah, right!"

"I don't know. Just happy. You kept saying neat things in your text; I thought you were a sensitive guy!"

The day came before I wanted it to. And how do I even begin to tell you what saying good-bye to Anthony was like? Early in the morning, Chelsea and I, with my car packed, followed Jimmy and Anthony in Jimmy's packed car, and made the trek to Virginia. With my brother also going back to Roanoke, there would be two good-byes in one. Jimmy's a pretty cool guy, and I would miss him as well.

It was weird for me, too. For the first time since I was very young, I wasn't going to school. I wasn't having that first-day "Felicia meeting." Even though it might be the same personnel at the school as the previous year, my parents and I always had to meet about my CF, either to reeducate new personnel or to update those who returned from the previous year.

Even though I was relieved not to have to study or get a paper in on time, I also felt a sense of loss. I loved learning. I wanted to continue some type of education, but I agreed with my parents that having been in and out of the hospital no less than eight times throughout high school, I did need a break.

Loss also came in hugging my friends good-bye. Fortunately, many of them, including Kelly and Nick, had chosen colleges in the area, so that lessened the trauma. In essence, regardless who'd be driving or flying off, my friends and I would still be hugging good-bye. But it was still hard to be the one turning around, heading home while they started new lives. My time to continue education would come–eventually.

As soon as we arrived at Roanoke, Chelsea and I helped the guys unpack and set up their rooms. We stayed a few days and then I couldn't delay the inevitable. The moment came to say good-bye to Anthony, a moment I wanted to disappear. I wished he went to college in Connecticut. But he didn't, and not all wishes come true.

I put on my strong face; I knew Anthony worried about being separated from me. We hugged and kissed and hugged and kissed. I'd approach the car and he'd inch toward it, too, leading to one more hug and one more kiss. Then, he'd turn and walk away. I'd run back to him–one more hug and kiss. I wouldn't see him for thirty-three days–until family weekend in October. It might as well have been a year.

As soon as Chelsea and I got on the highway heading home, I broke my don't-cry-in-front-of-other-people rule and burst into tears. Trying to hold back tears reminded me of that story I always loved about the boy in Holland and the dam. Chelsea spent the next thirty minutes consoling me. That finally helped me to stop crying. Then we turned the ride into a mini road trip, singing along loudly to songs on the radio, laughing and stopping at a truck stop for burgers and fries.

It was early evening when I dropped Chelsea off, hugged her good-bye, told her to say hello to Rory, and drove back to my house. She was starting her senior year of high school the next day, and I was starting something–yet to be determined.

Anthony was six hundred miles away, but the number of miles didn't matter. He wasn't holding my hand walking along the beach and looking for seashells, or cuddled next to me on a couch watching a movie, or lying beside me on a hammock and staring up at a starry night. He was at college, studying for a career in criminal justice. Other people got to see him every day, professors, roommates, classmates, the librarian, the checkout person at the bookstore–everyone but me.

Thirty-three days really wasn't a year. There I was, flying to Virginia with my father and stepmother for family weekend. I hugged Anthony and couldn't stop hugging him until Sunday night when another good-bye came way too soon and my father and stepmother took Chelsea's place as consoler for the ride home. Now it would be a stretch of almost seven weeks until Thanksgiving when I would see Anthony again. Or so I thought. Little did I know I would see him a lot sooner, but not for any reason I would have chosen.

Chapter Twelve

It was late at night and I was watching an episode of *Gilmore Girls*. It was one of the first shows from 2000 about Rory's first day going to Chilton Private School. As Rory and Lorelai drove toward the school, I thought the building in the background looked like the Goodspeed Opera House. I rewound the DVD, and it wasn't my imagination. Funny I never noticed this before, and I had watched this episode countless times. It gave me goose bumps and made me miss Anthony even more as I relived the day we went to the Goodspeed last summer. Even though it was almost the end of October, I still had twenty-four days before he'd be home for Thanksgiving. Although I'd be splitting my time between being with Anthony and going to my nana and papa's house for a family reunion from the Saturday before Thanksgiving until the Friday after, Anthony and I would still have one full day on the Saturday after Thanksgiving to be together. We had both agreed that that day would be just for us. Then it'd only be a few more weeks until winter break.

There would be no less than thirty family members gathering together Thanksgiving week. I had never missed a trip there except for that first hospitalization when I was in third grade. By now, my grandparents had retired to Aruba. Nana and Papa made the decision to move there with the stipulation that they treat all of us to a family reunion every year. There is nothing more important to my family than being together. Interestingly enough, this is a core value for Anthony's family as well. The Dellaripas value family time as much as I do.

When my papa was young, he started a small store for outdoor furniture in Connecticut. He believed in hard work and loyalty, and, eventually, he expanded to more and more stores and even opened stores in other states. But as he aged, he finally decided to retire, and he was fortunate to be able to gather us all together. Family and charity are the two most important places to spend money, my nana and papa always said. But sadly, he brought truth to the expression: money can't buy you health–not for Nana and not for me. That he had no greater power other than prayers.

This year especially, I was anxious to be with Nana. The last time we spoke on the phone, she sounded extremely frail. She told me she had developed a new complication in addition to her emphysema–MacLeod Syndrome, or MAC. This condition made it harder for her to breathe, and she was more susceptible to infections–similar to what I have with CF. That saddened me. Ever since I was a little girl, in addition to playing *Frustration* together, we shared our fears and frustrations about each other's medical conditions and consoled one another, whether in person or during the endless phone calls between us. The conversations just changed as I got older and I understood more about Nana and myself.

It was really late, but I knew Anthony was up studying. He had told me he would be earlier when we talked on the telephone, but I texted him so I wouldn't wake his roommate. I was excited to tell him about seeing the Goodspeed on this episode. Before I finished writing, I started to feel nauseous, really nauseous, and ended up throwing the cell phone on the bed as I ran to vomit. I freaked when I saw the toilet bowl filled with bright red liquid. As red as I've ever seen any blood. I screamed for my mother, who came running. She saw the horror on my face as I pointed to the red liquid swirling in the toilet bowl.

I could hardly understand Felicia, she was crying so hysterically. "I . . . vomit . . . blood . . . red . . . red . . . miss you . . . need you . . . hospital . . . ."

"Don't cry, Felicia. I'll be there. Please. Don't be scared. Yes, Jimmy will drive."

Ten minutes later, there we were, brother and boyfriend, driving through the night, heading north, book bags quickly thrown together along with a small duffle with barely a day's change of clothes. Toothbrushes could be bought later. No time to think of packing that.

I wasn't sure what to say to Jimmy about his sister, and I suspected he wasn't sure what to say to me about my girlfriend, so we just rode for a long time listening to the radio. Occasionally, I'd ask if he wanted me to drive. He assured me he'd let me know, which he did, and we stopped, traded places, and continued on our trek home to Connecticut to Felicia.

I often daydreamed of how I would handle a six on Felicia's cough rating scale. The night after I drove her home from our first date, after she gave me her rating system, I put 911 in my speed dial in my cell phone, as well as her mother's cell number, her father's, and Dr. P's emergency numbers.

But Felicia's hysterical phone call said she threw up blood. Nothing to do with coughing. This wasn't that dreaded number six in her rating system. I didn't have a plan for that. Why didn't I have a plan for that?

A few minutes after I took the wheel, Felicia's mother called to assure us that Felicia was fine. She had pancreatitis, an inflammation of the pancreas, and her doctor said she had to be on a liquid diet and also gave her some medicine, including one that made her sleepy.

Just as we entered Connecticut around six in the morning, Felicia's mother called again and told us to wait a few hours before coming to the hospital. Felicia was better, but still sleeping.

I called my parents so I wouldn't scare them if they heard me come in. My mother answered the phone and I explained what happened.

Jimmy dropped me off. I quietly opened the front door and tiptoed into the kitchen. My mother was waiting for me.

She silently hugged me, then pulled back. "I worry."

"She'll be OK."

"She's not the only one I worry about."

I had no answer, so I nodded, climbed the stairs to my room, picked up Rory, and sat in the dark with her on my lap. Then sleep took over.

So, I paid the consequences for my earlier rebellion against the enzymes that would have broken up the food to make it easier for me to digest. I continued a liquid diet for another two days plus my regular CF medicines and a new posthospital regimen.

Like my hospital stay the preceding June, Anthony sat with me all day, but instead of reading magazines or watching DVDs, he had his face in his books, trying to get his school work done. Although his professors had excused him from classes, Anthony didn't want to get behind in his studies. Besides, he didn't mind missing any *Gilmore Girls* episodes! Although, he confessed he was a bit curious to see the episode with the Goodspeed in it!

The last day of my hospital stay was Halloween. As soon as Dr. P checked me out to make sure I continued to be OK, I could be discharged. Because I was still in the pediatric section, we had a Halloween parade. Nurses and patients who were healthy enough marched up and down the hallways transformed into Batman, Spiderman, witches and princesses. After that, goody bags were distributed. One of the volunteers stopped at my bed and with a smile asked whether I was too old for a goody bag. I shook my head, smiled and took one. Like a kid after trick-or-treating, I dumped its contents on the bed and had fun sorting through all the trinkets and candy.

Later that day, shortly before I was discharged, Anthony and Jimmy showed up with *their* goody bag filled with coloring books and crayons, and Chelsea brought me a tiara and a wand to dress up like a princess. I put on the tiara and I did feel like a princess.

Anthony had one other surprise, a real treat. He had officially applied to transfer to Western Connecticut State University (WCSU) here in Connecticut, not in Virginia. Another type of medicine to help me get better.

Actually, he had been tossing around this idea for a few weeks, no longer sure of what he wanted to major in, not sure whether he and Roanoke College were still a good match. Plus he wanted to be close to home for a variety of reasons. (I came under that category!)

After three days in the hospital, I was discharged and the next morning, I watched Jimmy and Anthony–after an inordinate amount of hugs, kisses and thank yous–back out of the driveway to return to school. Then I turned and went in the house to start my breathing machine and chest percussions. I began a new countdown of three weeks before all the exciting events around Thanksgiving.

But the second week of November, my mom gave me a piece of news that sent me into a fury that went well beyond the anger I felt two years ago when I was told I needed a lung transplant. Until now, my nana and I both were able to be with one another because her emphysema and my CF were not contagious diseases. Someone with a compromised immune system, i.e., me, on the other hand, could pick up MAC.

When I was six years old, I cultured pseudonomas. It stays in the lungs and colonizes for the rest of my life. I can never get rid of it. It traps infections, making it harder for me to get better. It is also contagious and dangerous, not only to other

CF patients, but to anyone with a weakened immune system such as paraplegics, AIDS, hepatitis patients, and anyone with a respiratory disease. This was another one of my mother's concerns for me to be with Nana.

In the end, it was far too dangerous for me to be with her. MAC is one of those bacterial infections, like pseudonomas, that is difficult, if not impossible, for CF patients to recover from. These types of bacterial infections become resistant to oral antibiotics and, eventually, to IV antibiotics as well. Translated, I couldn't go to the reunion.

This time I knew exactly where to direct my fury. Straight at CF. I knew I'd get nowhere arguing with my mother. She told me she had given this a great deal of thought and if I caught MAC, I'd be in real danger. I was also warned that I would probably have another bout of pancreatitis. I didn't care about that. Being with Nana was way more important. But my mother wouldn't let me go.

My CF forced me to grow up long before I was ready to. I knew that defying my mother and trying to go see Nana regardless of our health issues would not have been responsible at all. If I contracted MAC and my health failed, how would that make Nana feel? And if I took this reality check one step further, there was no way Nana, because she loved me, would have let me visit her and jeopardize my health. I knew only too well by now what effects my actions or choices about my health had on the people I love.

Thus, without the intense arguments of two years ago, I simply resigned myself to not going. That was the responsible and only possible decision. I was frustrated, angry, sad, and, worse, mean to my mom, something I was very rarely. My mother has made many sacrifices because of and for me. Although I could have gone to my dad's for Thanksgiving and stayed with him while she and Jimmy flew down to be with the family, my mother insisted she would stay home with me and visit her parents a few weeks later. She also offered me a trip to New York City for a few days, to shop, eat, see the Macy's Thanksgiving Day parade. They were both generous offers, but, at the time, they seemed a paltry substitute. I continued to be nasty to her for not letting me go on the trip. My heart refused to listen to my head.

As I withdrew into myself from this major disappointment, I recognized another aspect of my world that was far different than two years ago. Anthony was now in my life, and, unfortunately, I also made him the target of my behavior, but in a different way. I became detached. This detachment led to my first authentic fight with Anthony.

Two people whom I needed the most right now and I couldn't have acted worse toward them. And that made my life even worse.

All events with Anthony are significant, but first-time events hold a different place in my heart: first date; first time he held my hand; first dance/sway; first kiss; called me girlfriend; and put in my IV antibiotics; so, too, will I always remember our first argument.

The first inkling of this fight could not have come at a poorer time. But then again, is there ever a good time? Or did I truly believe I would have a deep relationship with him and never have a disagreement? Anthony immediately picked up on my apathetic tone at the onset of our first conversation after I learned of my plight.

He asked what was wrong.

"Nothing."

He asked again.

"Nothing."

Of all the times that I needed him to comfort me the most, even long-distance from Virginia, I wouldn't let him in. My conversations with him became only clipped answers as I crawled deeper into myself.

One of the benefits of not getting on the plane with the rest of the family should have been the chance to spend more time with Anthony, but I had mixed feelings. Excited to spend time with him, I was also angry I wasn't with my nana and the rest of the family and distraught in my shutdown mode. So when he came home from college on the Monday before Thanksgiving and I was still in Connecticut, I got what should have been bonus days. But all that brought were more clipped answers, more refusals to explain why I wasn't on the trip–in person instead of in e-mails, texts or telephone calls. I didn't share this fight with my mother, father or friends. That, too, I kept to myself.

"Look, Felicia, if we are going to be a couple, you need to talk to me." Those were Anthony's words that Monday night. After two hours of either silence or short answers to his questions, Anthony was angry with me.

"Hey, Felicia, want to watch . . . ?"

"I don't care."

"Rather go out?"

"Whatever you want."

"Are you OK?"

"Fine, Anthony, just fine."

"Something wrong?"

"No."

"There's something wrong. I can tell."

"Anthony, if there were something wrong, I'd tell you."

Right. Nothing was wrong. Felicia just wouldn't talk to me. I was really getting angry. This was turning into much more than what we had labeled the "annoyance" when she texted that old boyfriend over the summer. I didn't like this feeling, and her sharp tone was really beginning to get to me.

Felicia sometimes gets in moods when she doesn't want to talk to anyone. That's OK. I just need a warning. In the past, if Felicia was frustrated or angry about something, she'd go to sleep and it would be gone the next day. But this missed trip to Aruba seemed to take more than one night's sleep. What made it hard for me was that I am the type of person who needs to talk things out, like that text the first night we began to correspond.

How was I going to help her if she didn't allow me in to her life?

Later in the evening, Anthony called and said he had a favor. That whatever was bothering me, could I just communicate with him somehow.

"Like, just say, 'mood' but don't not talk to me without telling me why."

I got the double negative, and I spoke in a less clipped way as I agreed to those terms. His temporary solution soothed me.

My mother and I arrived in the city early Tuesday afternoon. We checked into the hotel and decided to rest before hitting the shops. I leaned my head on her shoulder and tried not to think of Anthony and our fight but wasn't having much success. Although the argument didn't still have the same intensity, it wasn't resolved, either. My mother stroked my hair.

"You know what I just thought of? The most ironic thing. I never even connected it until now. When you were a little girl, do you remember refusing to go to your dad's for Thanksgiving because I'd be alone? How ironic. Now the situation's reversed."

My mother shook her head in disbelief.

"I'm sorry I've been so awful," I said quietly.

"I know you are."

She continued to stroke my hair.

We bundled up, walked up and down the avenues, and shopped while we nibbled on hot roasted peanuts bought from a street vendor. On Thursday morning, we feasted on a special Thanksgiving brunch, headed out to watch the Macy's Day Parade, and returned home, having added more special mother/daughter memories. On the way home, I repeatedly thanked my mother for a great Thanksgiving, even though I was still sad about the turn in events.

I also announced, "And when Nana gets better, I'll be able to go see her."

By late afternoon, we were back home, and my mother asked if I wanted to go to Anthony's house. I knew by now that his family had eaten their Thanksgiving dinner. I only had until Sunday morning to be with him before he drove back to college, and it was time to let him know why I had been so upset.

Two simple sentences. One explaining why I couldn't be with Nana, the other to apologize for my behavior.

"What? Contagious? I mean, that sucks. I mean, I'm sorry, Felicia."

I explained and I sobbed. Really sobbed. He held me in his arms, stroked my hair, comforting me until the tears finally subsided.

"If we are going to be in a relationship, I want you when you are happy, when you are sad, when you are angry, have a ketchup spill on your shirt, have a ketchup spill on my shirt and–"

Spontaneously our hands reached for each other. The fight was over. This certainly wasn't in the same category as the one about me texting while Anthony and I watched a movie. I called it a fight because you don't have to scream or yell to define something as a "fight," like when my mother and I had screamed about the whole meds and transplant thing. To Anthony and me, a fight was a serious difference of opinion, whether we shouted at each other or I withdrew and didn't talk. As in so many other aspects of our relationship, once we resolved it, our relationship grew deeper, stronger, and we were more accepting of each other.

Although we patched up our differences, a dark cloud still lingered over my excitement of being with Anthony. I was still in Connecticut and missed being with my nana and the rest of the family for the reunion.

Laura's Journal

Ever since I was a little girl, long before I married or became Jimmy and Felicia's mom, I always thought death was the final gift of life. Watching *my* mom, now stricken with MAC, struggle for each breath confirmed that thought. That was something a daughter never wants to see a parent have to go through, and something a parent never wants to see a child go through. Gasping, struggling, the fear of not breathing; seeing death walk closer.

They say mothers and fathers today often become part of a "sandwich" generation, take care of their children and take care of their parents at the same time. It's a very odd feeling, watching my past and my future go through similar struggles, knowing all the while I'm alone in the middle. I was wedged between two choices, to be with my ailing mother whose time on this Earth was of short measure or to be with a disappointed

daughter for a holiday while her time on this
Earth was . . . .

What a position to be in.

Anthony and I spent the rest of Thanksgiving evening, all day
Friday, Saturday, and one hour of Sunday morning together
before he had to drive back to school. These few days were
magical reminders of the carefree summer days we had shared.
Yet they were frantic days as we tried not only to have fun but
also to somehow make up for time lost fighting. So despite my
sadness at not seeing my family, my mood improved.

One week after the Thanksgiving break, my brother called
from school with an idea for Anthony's birthday in early
December. I listened to the details and couldn't think of a better
birthday present.

Anthony's birthday came on a Tuesday that year, and Jimmy
told me his fraternity was throwing him a big bash the Saturday
before. Not a surprise to Anthony, just a big party.

Now here's the best part. Jimmy didn't have any classes
on Fridays and of the two he had on Thursday, one was
canceled and one was an independent project due just before
reading period for exams began. He planned to drive to
Connecticut Wednesday night to be with his girlfriend, who
lived up here. When he put the whole calendar together and
realized the party was Saturday night, he suggested I drive
back with him and surprise Anthony. Then I could stay and
drive back home with Anthony after finals. Jimmy knew that
I loved exploring life and would find plenty of things to do. I
wouldn't be bored, even though I couldn't spend much time
with Anthony while he studied and took finals–except for a
little celebration on his actual birthday! What a plan! First,
though, I asked Jimmy who I ask about an invitation because
I wouldn't want to go where I wasn't invited. He said he
already took care of it. With that cleared, I put my plan into

action. First on the list of to dos was to shop for the biggest bow I could find.

The night of the party, with a bight red bow that covered my whole shirt, I waited in a corner behind a door in the living room of his fraternity house. When Anthony came down from his bedroom, Jimmy motioned him over to talk to him. Then, after the shock that I was standing there wore off, he gave *me* a surprise of a lifetime! That very day the letter had come from WSCU. He was accepted as a transfer student! He was waiting for the perfect way to surprise me with the news, and I had unexpectedly supplied that way.

For the next few days, I took pictures, sketched jewelry, read books, and waited for Anthony to take his last final exam before we drove home. This drive back to Connecticut was far different than the others I had taken earlier in the fall. This time, no good-byes, no tears, no need for consolers. I sat next to Anthony and smiled the whole way home.

For the next few weeks, we spent time shopping for gifts, wrapping them while listening to carols, baking sugar cookies that I taught Anthony how to decorate, and attending numerous holiday parties. With the start of a new year, my calendar would no longer be a series of Xs until Anthony finally came home.

Chapter Thirteen

The Monday in January just before the new semester started at WCSU, Anthony and I were playing a game of *Frustration*. I had taught it to him, Nana's version. It was a gloomy, dreary day. The snow wasn't pretty like when it first falls and is fresh and pure white, or my favorite, when it decorates the trees converting bare branches into picture postcards. Anthony got up to get a can of Monster, asked if I wanted anything to drink. I shook my head no. When he came back to the den, he stopped at the window and stared out at the gray day as dusk settled in and turned the gray into black.

Suddenly he turned and said, "Let's go out."

"Now? It's so yucky and cold out."

"I know."

Fifteen minutes later we were seated at Bill's with our baskets of food and the band started its first set of the evening. Anthony and I stepped onto the dance floor and swayed to the music.

Three days later, Anthony started his next semester of school, this time only eighty miles away. Not six hundred.

Eighty. My weekends were going to be a lot happier than when he was in Virginia. We would alternate me going there and him coming back to Old Saybrook. Somehow I'd survive the days in between.

For the next four months nothing extraordinary happened. Let me rephrase that. Each day of life is extraordinary. By nothing I mean no midnight scares of bloody vomit, no bronchs, and no collapsed lung forcing difficult choices. Sometime in those four months, I finally stopped worrying about Anthony being overwhelmed by me. He'd seen some pretty severe aspects of my life with CF and, each time, surprised me how much he could handle.

While still not happy about not being able to hug Nana, I made the best of what I could. She and I continued our special relationship by phone, e-mail, and exchanging special greeting cards. And because my papa wouldn't leave Nana as her condition worsened, I missed him as well. I still clung to a thread of hope that Nana would get better. I daydreamed of getting on a plane and running into her arms. We'd hug and play more games of *Frustration*. But that was never to be. Three months later my nana died. I never saw her again. Never got to hug her, feel her strong hands around me as she told me I brought her sunshine.

And then it was one year since our first date. Anthony's plan to celebrate our anniversary was to cook dinner for me at his house. He asked to have the kitchen and dining room for ourselves, and his parents agreed. He picked me up, brought me into his house and the smell of garlic permeated the kitchen. He said dinner was ready and escorted me into the dining room. The table was set with a white tablecloth, fine china, candles, and a flower centerpiece. It looked so romantic, I gasped. But Anthony stood there perplexed. I asked what was wrong. He shrugged and said that he had set the table before leaving to pick me up, but this was not how it looked. We later found out that the same loving culprit who secretly told the waiters at Max Downtown to say happy birthday to me almost a year ago, had rearranged Anthony's table setting because he didn't do it correctly! He shook his head in amazement and said he was lucky to have such a cool mother.

Anthony pulled out my chair. I sat and he disappeared briefly before returning with a platter of chicken parmigiana and pasta. He lit the candles and said we needed some music to accompany our dinner. He turned on his Ipod in the speaker docking station. I smiled as Nat King Cole's *Unforgettable* came on. I swear, sometimes I think I'm living a fantasy in a romance novel. How romantic and sweet to put this song on his Ipod and play it for our dinner. The next song was *Mona Lisa*, also a Nat King Cole tune. This was followed by *Stardust,* and I finally asked, "Just how many of his songs did you put on your Ipod?"

"All of them."

The songs were still playing when we finished dinner and Anthony stood up and asked me to dance. He asked me! What a difference a year makes! Hard to believe a simple text that started out with having no idea who was writing to me turned into this magical relationship. So right there in the middle of the dining room, we swayed to Nat King Cole.

All evening long, I had the sense that Anthony wanted to say something more that what he was saying. A couple of times, he started a sentence with "um, ah, I" and then stopped and said something related to the dinner or what song was playing, but it seemed like that wasn't what he really meant. Did he have another surprise for me?

After dinner, we lay on the hammock just as we had first done a year ago. We were quiet until I found Orion's Belt. We decided to share anything we wanted about our first year together, what attracted us to each other or what we have learned about each other over the year.

I went first. I told Anthony that I liked how he stays dedicated and committed to something if he is passionate about it and how he takes good care of it. Like drumming. When I say he takes good care of it, I mean more than just making sure the drums are in good condition and keeping that area of his makeshift disco clean and uncluttered. That's a given. I mean he takes good care of the passion. He and the drums are one. I realized that the passion grew over the year. He seemed to slow down and savor the drumming, be in the moment, the way I tried to teach him from our very first date. And not be worried about the next step of his life after he finished playing. I felt good I could be his teacher.

Although it wasn't something new in the past year, I reminded him how I love to listen to him play drums and I never get bored. I adore the drums and I adore Anthony, so the combination still amazes me.

I also shared how I liked that he was never afraid to show his feelings, right from when he admitted on our first date that he was scared to go on a roller coaster. He is himself.

Then it was his turn to tell me.

"How adorable you are," he blurted out.

I blushed.

"Seriously, and not just that. You are so polite and kind toward me, and as our relationship grew, you learned not to be afraid to let me have my guy time."

I nodded, remembering the first few times he said he was busy and going out with the guys. I thought I had done something wrong. Eventually, I came to understand that, yes, we have a relationship and are a couple, yet we each have our lives, and those individual lives are what also enhanced our relationship.

"When was your first date?" Anthony suddenly asked.

"*My* first date? I don't remember, maybe seventh or eighth

grade. It was very profound. A boy would say, 'I like you,' and I'd say, 'I like you' and then we'd hold hands in the hallways changing classes."

"No, I mean a real date."

I remember my first-date jitters, and they had nothing do with CF. Just being alone with a boy without a group of friends around. He knew I had CF. I knew I had CF. But that fact never entered my mind that night, from the moment I got in the back seat of his mother's car, through the entire movie and to the moment he got out of my mom's car later!

"Let's see. The first time my mom let me go out with a boy by myself, I was nervous because it wasn't a hand-holding walk in the school hallway with tons of other kids and teachers around. It was just the two of us. We went to the movies. His mom drove and my mom picked us up. I remember, it was Christmastime and we exchanged these little gifts. Gawd, that seems like a century ago! And your first date?"

"Just a girl I met at school and asked to the movies. Seventh grade as well. It was all so new, going out with a girl."

Anthony suddenly leaned over and gave me a kiss–long, warm, and tender–and I responded the same way. Long, warm, tender–and cough-free.

He pulled back and smiled.

"Happy Anniversary."

"Happy Anniversary."

When I opened my anniversary gift, I couldn't stop laughing, crying, and hugging him. I held two tickets for a day's admission to Six Flags Amusement Park. So that was why he must have been hesitating so much, waiting for the right moment to give me the gift. Or at least that was my assumption.

I pointed to the huge gift I left on the counter when I came in and told him to open it. His enthusiasm for his gift matched mine. It was a large jar I had filled with 365 pieces of paper, each with different ways he made me feel, one to read each day for the upcoming year. Anthony had given me a future.

Three days later, I turned nineteen. For my birthday, my friend Daniela called and said Anthony wanted her to pick me up and bring me to a restaurant. He'd be waiting there. He couldn't get home from his summer job–this year at a mini-golf place–in time to shower, change, pick me up, and get to the restaurant at a decent hour. So he asked Daniela and her boyfriend if they could help out. And my only instructions were to bring a sweater because he arranged for outdoor seating. One other request. Anthony asked Daniela to blindfold me so I wouldn't know where I was going until I got there. Everything went off on time. Daniela and her boyfriend picked me up. I got in the car, carrying a white cardigan. Daniela put on the blindfold and started to drive. I think she made a few extra turns because there was no way I could figure out where we were going. She finally stopped the car, helped me out of it, walked me to the pavement, and stopped. She said that we were here and I could take off my blindfold. As I pulled it off, the word, "Surprise" was shouted at me as I saw I was in Anthony's backyard about to step on the lawn where twenty friends stood, including Anthony and Nick, who stood side by side, grinning ear to ear. They had teamed up to surprise me and had engaged Daniela and her boyfriend to help carry out the plan.

The yard was covered with balloons. A Slip n' Slide was set up as well as an area to play bocce. And food was everywhere. Chips, salsa, my favorite hummus, cheese and crackers, vegetable platter, sodas. A large bowl of summer fruit and of course, a birthday cake with purple roses.

I was in awe. "You guys did this?"

Anthony and Nick slung their arms around each other and nodded like proud little boys who had behaved in school. I was so happy Anthony and Nick had connected. Kind of like Chelsea and I had bonded. After all, Nick was like a brother to me, someone I'd spent almost every day of my life with growing up, having lived next door to one another; Nick, who used to take me to look for golf balls in the woods near our house. Nick, who liked to make me laugh and who, one time when we were little and went on a picnic, said something silly while I was drinking water. I laughed and I spurted the water all over his shirt, soaking it to the point where he ran home screaming, "Cooties, Cooties." Nick, who was at the hospital and held my hand for an hour and cried when Dr. P said my lung had partially collapsed. Nick, who saw how my mother and I struggled with the chest percussion vest and machine and suggested a special cart, and who within one day measured the machine and, with his dad's help, constructed a custom-made cart that made it easier for us to move the machine. Nick, who has told me that someday, when he gets married, I will be in his wedding as the best "woman" or some other special role.

When Anthony came into my life, he and I, along with Nick and his girlfriend, went out together or if Nick wasn't seeing anyone steadily or didn't have a date, the three of us would go to a movie, dinner, miniature golf, whatever. And as the weeks passed and Anthony became a more and more important part of my life, he embraced Nick as a special person in my life and Nick and Anthony became friends–first because they had me in common, and, eventually, they developed their own friendship. They'd go out and do something they both liked. Yes, Nick, who will be my friend forever, and Anthony, who will hopefully always be in my life, planned this cool surprise party.

Then there was their "accomplice" Daniela–a true friend,

someone who has always stood by me as well. An always-there-for-me friend. She'd find me wherever I was, in the hospital, at home sick, in school, and always made sure I was OK. And if I wasn't, she'd find out why, then search for the answer to try to make me OK. She was a giver and taker. She helped me but didn't refuse my help when she needed it. I loved that about her. She never said, "Felicia, you have enough to deal with." If she was bummed out, she listened to my advice, allowed me to drive her to someone's house or do an errand for her if I offered.

Just as Anthony was lighting the candles for the cake, his brother Andrew came over to me and whispered, "I know with me at college and stuff, I don't get to see you much, but I want to let you know, you're a cool kid. And, ah, I've never seen my brother so happy with a girl."

I gave Andrew a hug and then took Anthony's hand as I blew out my candles. They say it's bad luck to tell what you wished for, so I won't. But I will let you know what I wished for one year ago on my eighteenth birthday because it already came true–that I would celebrate my nineteenth birthday.

Chapter Fourteen

"You ready?"

"Yes."

"Anthony, we don't have to do this."

"Yes, we do. You said I was going on the biggest and scariest one for my roller coaster inauguration and I am."

"I know, but if you want to start on a smaller one than *Superman,* it's OK."

"When have you ever known me not to plunge head first into something?"

I had no argument for someone who started my medical care by visiting me at the hospital everyday, staying up for three weeks to insert medicine into a pic line, then went on a doctor's appointment. That isn't exactly building up slowly. Besides, he stood firm that he was going to trust me about a roller coaster ride.

So we finally made it to an amusement park and to Anthony's first roller coaster. In truth, I think I was equally nervous for Anthony, if not more so. If he hated it, being stuck up there for the couple of minutes that the ride lasted could feel like forever.

I took a sip of water and used my inhaler before putting the water bottle and inhaler back in my pocketbook and shoving it into the locker provided for the roller coaster riders. I handed Anthony the key to hold, then handed over our tickets, boarded the ride, where we strapped ourselves in, and waited for the ride to start. I looked to Anthony and tried to interpret his feelings. I patted his hand that he'd be fine and could trust me.

"Don't worry. You'll be with me. Once you get over the first drop, it's fun. Like a huge adrenalin rush."

He nodded as the ride started. I knew exactly when the first big drop would come, so I kept my eyes focused on Anthony and hoped he'd laugh and not freak. The car took that steep dip. Anthony laughed! I laughed! Whew!

The ride ended and he couldn't stop thanking me, almost jumping up and down as he babbled something about where has something this phenomenal been hiding all these years? We grabbed our belongings and plunked ourselves down on a bench to pick out the next rides. We figured there'd be enough time for three more rides before the concert at the amusement park, included in Anthony's anniversary gift. He wanted to know my favorite roller coaster rides to choose, but I told him all of them and that he should pick. He figured it out from the biggest and scariest down to the smallest as well as different kinds. So after *Superman*, he decided on *Batman*, *Scream* and last–*Cyclone,* one of the older and smaller roller coasters. I assured him all were good choices–I'd been on them all hundreds of times.

Like little kids, hand in hand, we ran from ride to ride; Anthony loved each one more and more. While I didn't expect to have everything in common with him, as I had discovered over the past year, riding roller coasters was something I was so happy we now could share. It was becoming quickly apparent how much Anthony loved them. The rides were so much more exciting with Anthony beside me.

We got off *Scream* and headed to *Cyclone.* Just as we had

for the other three rides, we threw our belongings in the locker, boarded the ride and strapped ourselves in. As we waited for the ride to start, Anthony declared that the next time we came back to the amusement park, we'd have to come earlier so we could try the rest of the roller coasters. Sounded good to me.

The first drop came. We both looked at each other and screamed in delight, but as my back was thrown against the seat, something happened: I couldn't breathe. Big time. I started to cough and gasp for breath. I knew right away this was bad, very bad. Maybe a number six bad.

I clutched Anthony's arm to try and reposition my body, but as the roller coaster sped up and down and took sharp corners, it was virtually impossible to do anything but sit strapped into the car as I coughed and gasped. The look on Anthony's face was devastating as he desperately tried to wrangle his body and shouted to the ground for help, but his desperate cries were lost in the wind and screams of the riders. He flagged his hands toward the ground and continued to call for help as I continued to gasp for breath.

Chapter Fifteen

The ride was over.

Anthony and I were still suspended in the air as each car moved toward the exit. Anthony continued to shout, but I stopped him as my coughing slowed down and my breathing became less labored. The car pulled up to the exit gate. Anthony helped me out of the car, sat me down on a bench, and bolted to the locker to get my pocketbook. Within a minute he was running back to me, water bottle and inhaler in hand, and sat down next to me. Although I felt OK by this point, I used the inhaler and gulped some water. Anthony jumped up and paced agitatedly, wiping tears from his eyes.

"How can you act so calm? You couldn't breathe. You almost died up there."

"I'm fine now. Calm down. Please. I don't know how else to tell you. I'm OK. My body slammed against the seat and suddenly I was coughing and gasping for breath."

I was devastated that I made him freak. Yet this was my life and maybe it was better he saw the worst of it now. Or what was the worst at this point. Who knows how bad my health could get? This was as close to a number six as I had ever had. Was this my test of how much reality could he handle? What was his saturation point? The calm I had started to feel a few months ago about Anthony being able to date me *and* handle CF and all its baggage rapidly disappeared.

I braced for Anthony's "I thought I could do this but I can't" speech. I actually felt myself physically pressing my legs against the bench as I prepared myself for the words. Then I realized the right thing to do was to save *him* the agony of the speech and let him bow out with dignity. As agonizing as it was, I needed to break off the relationship and say good-bye. I always believed in not being afraid to get my feet wet, to go after dreams and goals. I knew I had tried this relationship with Anthony and it hadn't worked. I tried to comfort myself by taking the positive approach. I had a phenomenal year with someone I . . . I realized that my next thought was . . . with someone I loved. Someone I loved! Somewhere along the line, I had fallen in love with Anthony. I was so stunned by my realization.

How could this have happened to me? How could I even tell him that I love him? I had to be strong. I also knew that loving a person means being selfless and always taking the other person's feelings into account, especially when making tough decisions. And it's not like I haven't had any experience in tough decision making in the past. I knew what I had to do, what the right thing to do was.

It was so noisy; I bent my head toward his so he could hear me better. My eyes started to well up with tears, but that uncanny skill of holding back tears served me well then. I'd cry privately later.

"If you don't want to be in a relationship with me, I'll understand."

"I love you," Anthony blurted out.

My mouth dropped open. We stared at one another speechless.

The silence continued until I smiled and whispered back, "I love you, too."

And despite the noise of the roller coaster taking its next group of people out to scream in delight, Anthony took me in his arms and nodded that he heard my words.

And I cried with happiness.

Epilogue

I realized that day at the amusement park that I had no idea what kind of a ride I was in for when I started to date Felicia. How ironic. How metaphoric. And not just any ride. A roller coaster. Ups and down, dips and climbs. All I knew is that I loved her.

I also realized I had really fallen in love with Felicia a year ago, only a few weeks after we started to date. I can pinpoint the exact moment. We were sitting in the Goodspeed Opera House to see Singing in the Rain. *I sat there in awe of how she was so engrossed in the dance and the music. Twenty minutes before she had given in to a what if? moment about the possibility of the tickets conflicting with her bronch. Then she jumped into enjoying–truly enjoying–the musical. I remember finding myself looking at her more than the actors on stage, and something changed in me. I had wondered if it could be love. I mean I liked her so much and was so happy when we were together, but I dismissed it, thinking I was nineteen and what did I know at that age and after only dating her a month. What did I know about real love? But I did know. And it was love. I tried to tell her my feelings at our anniversary dinner a few days earlier before our* trip to the amusement park, tell her how much I loved her, but I couldn't quite find the words.

I knew our relationship could survive anything, because I had respect for Felicia and she for me. Without that respect, I don't think any relationship can work.

So I loved her unconditionally, through all of the hospital visits, fights, bad mood days and anything else that comes our way.

When I look at Felicia, CF doesn't automatically come into my mind; that was one of the biggest surprises in dating her. I thought I would constantly think about it. One day, it occurred to me that I never thought about it except when it applied to what we were doing in the moment or making plans. And there were two Felicias in my life; at least two different mindsets of Felicia. Felicia with cystic fibrosis and Felicia without cystic fibrosis. The first time I became aware of that concept was a year ago when we bought the rabbit. I guess I was thinking about the rabbit in my non-CF mindset. And if I were to continue having this beautiful young woman in my life, I would have to find a way to mesh the two, if at all possible. But I truly, deeply, unquestionably loved her, and doesn't love conquer all?

People who know about Felicia and her lung transplant issue all ask me the same question, "Why don't you talk Felicia into a lung transplant so you'll have a better chance of a life together?" And I give the same answer. I just try to encourage her to do what she feels is best for herself, because I never want to see her suffer or be unhappy, no matter what the cost.

I sat on the bench next to Felicia at the amusement park, her hand safely tucked into mine, and more thoughts jumped through my mind, including some of my own what ifs? What if Emily hadn't annoyed me that night at the ball game? I might not have been looking for someone else to talk to. What if I hadn't organized the address book in my cell phone by first names? Or, what if I knew other girls whose names started with the letters A to E? I might have texted one of them.

I also thought about how Felicia came into my life when it

was hectic with college and studying as well as at a time when I questioned everything, like what I would do with the rest of my life. She brought a sense of comfort and peace to me. She is my best friend, someone I take care of and someone who takes care of me. Until Felicia, I had brushed a lot of life aside, unlike Felicia, who lives every day to its fullest. I was so concerned about my future, I forgot to live day by day. We are each other's teacher and we are in love. How thankful–and lucky–I am.

I have no idea what the future holds. No one does, really, if you think about it. No one knows the very next second. If my mother's trip hadn't been canceled on that September day in 2001, and she had boarded that plane, her life would have turned out differently. Some people have more of an idea about life than others. I've figured that out, too. Felicia has had some cold, hard facts to deal with. As I also do by being in love with her. I love her and never want her out of my sight, no matter how long we have together–or don't have. And if that means giving up things, I will. I know how easily Felicia can slip away. Hey, I could have lost her there on that roller coaster while the rest of the riders were screaming with joy, giggling, enjoying the moment, seemingly without a care in the world. Something as simple as a ride on a roller coaster could knock the wind out of her. But as Felicia has taught me, all we have is the present. So right now, I'm going to have fun with my girlfriend, hanging out at the amusement park.

Next on the list of having fun? Check out the concession stand for some Sour Patch Kids–and we'll pick out the red and the green ones together.

Breathing Machine

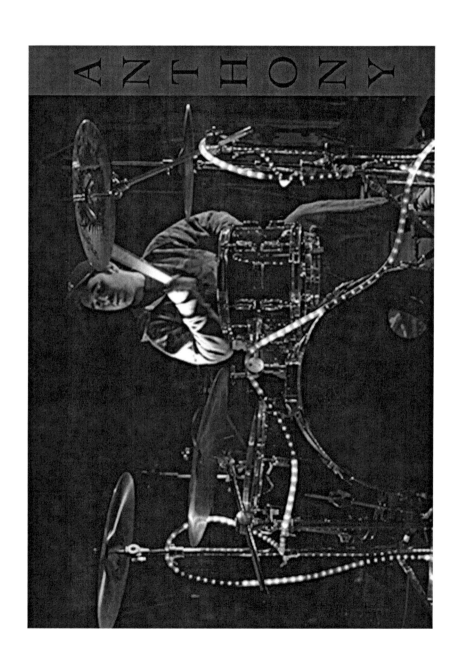

ANTHONY

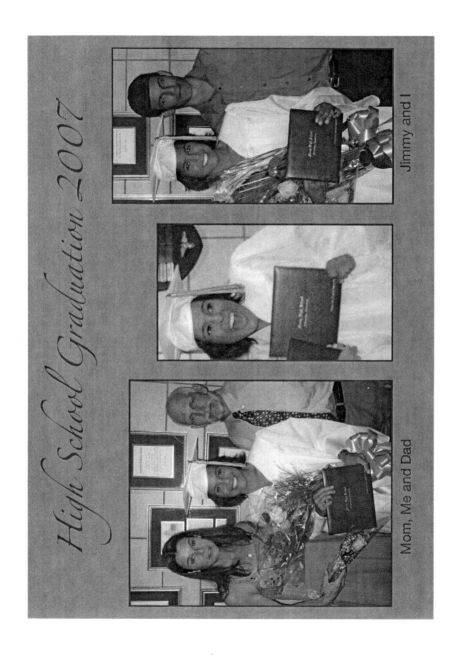

High School Graduation 2007

Jimmy and I

Mom, Me and Dad

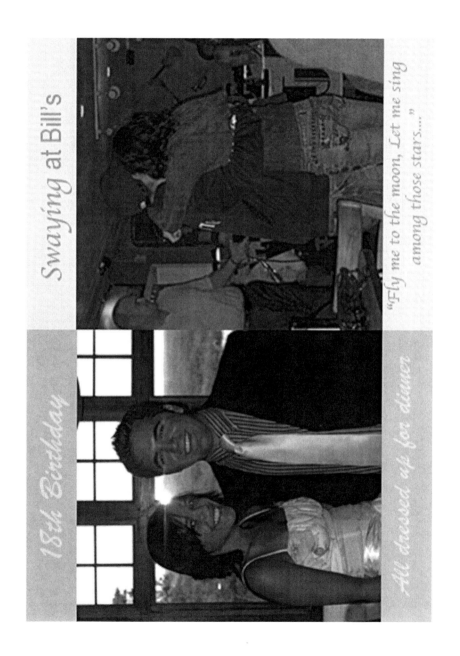

Swaying at Bill's

"Fly me to the moon, Let me sing among those stars...."

18th Birthday

All dressed up for dinner

SASHA BABY

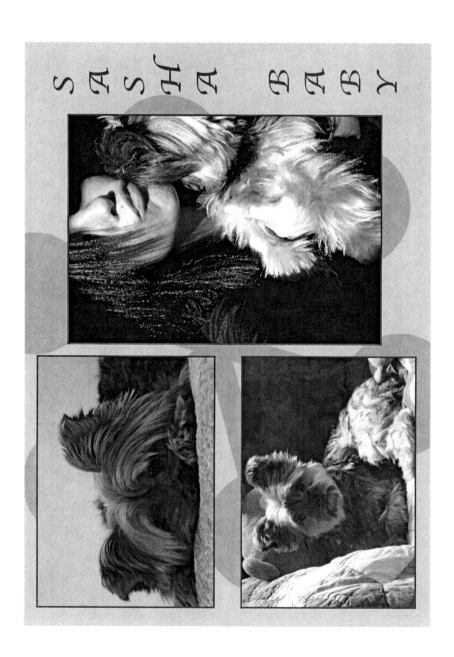

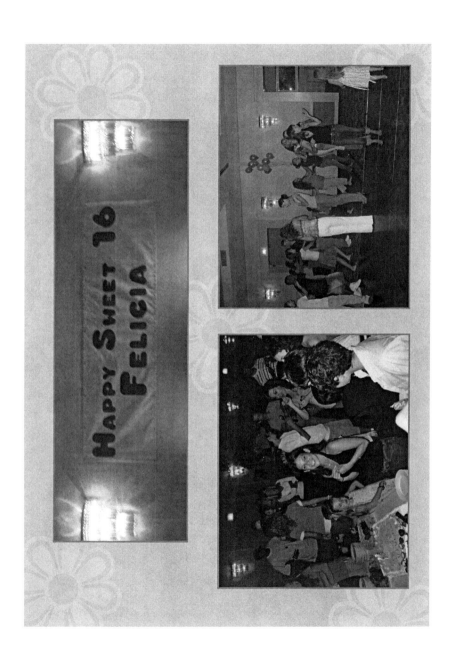

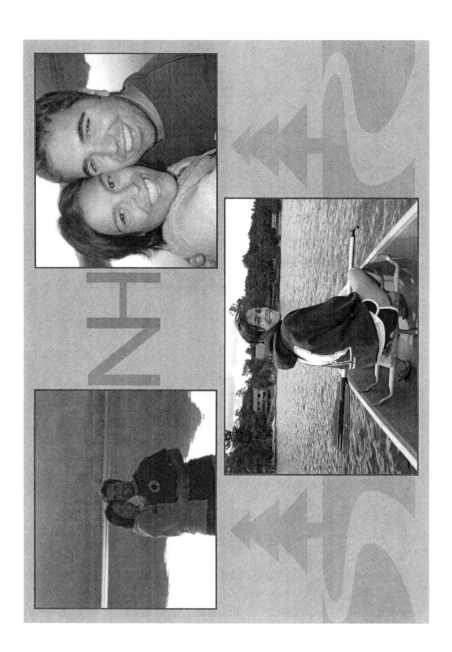

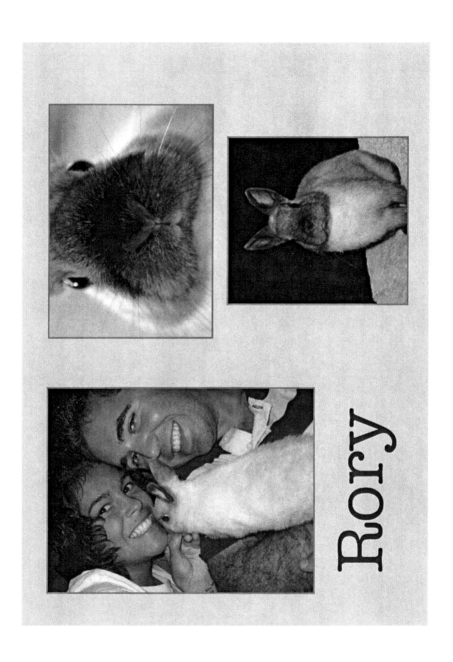

Rory

Nana & Papa

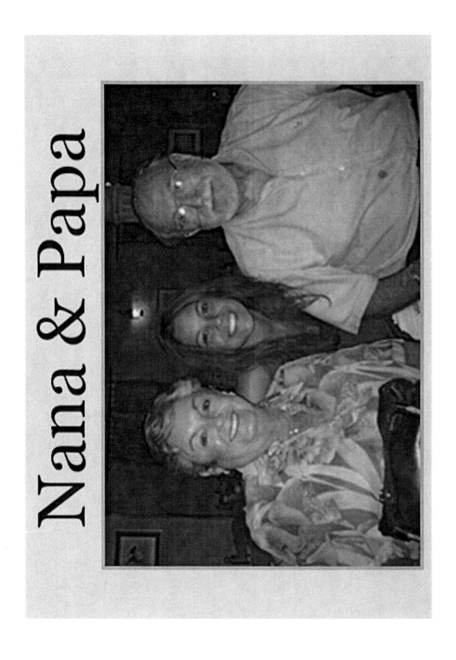

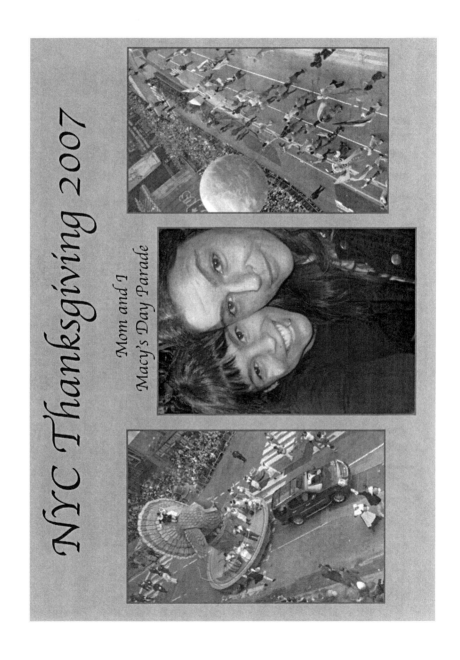

NYC Thanksgiving 2007

Mom and I
Macy's Day Parade

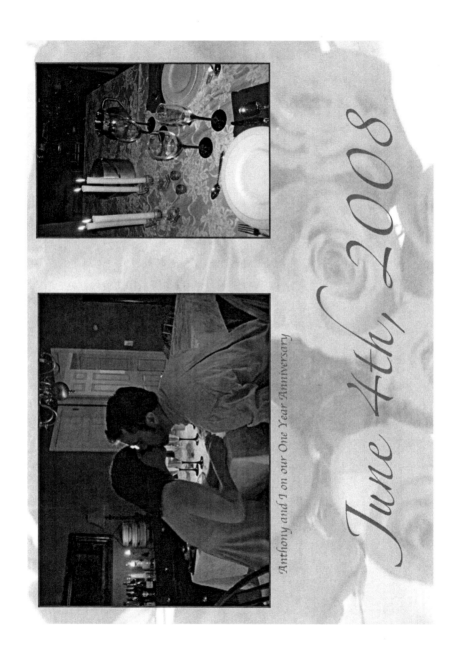

Anthony and I on our One Year Anniversary

June 4th, 2008

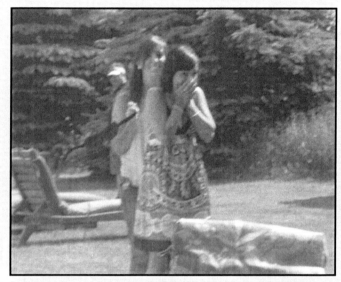

Surprise!!

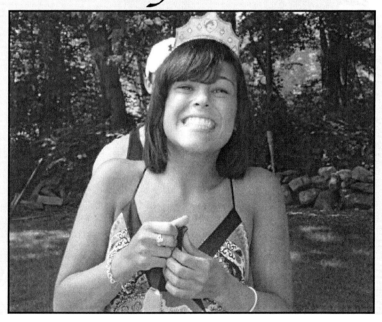

SIX FLAGS

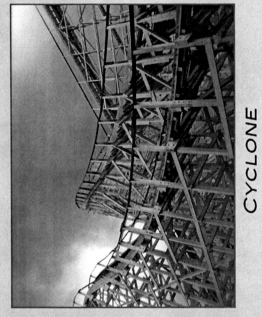

CYCLONE

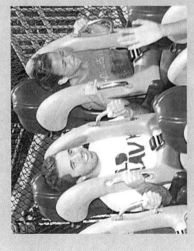

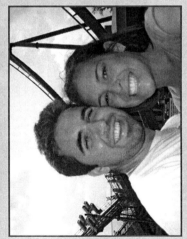

The Girls!

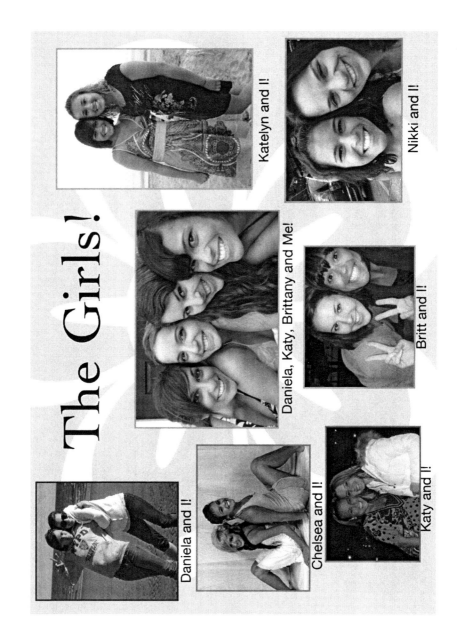

Katelyn and I!

Nikki and I!

Daniela, Katy, Brittany and Me!

Britt and I!

Daniela and I!

Chelsea and I!

Katy and I!

The Boys

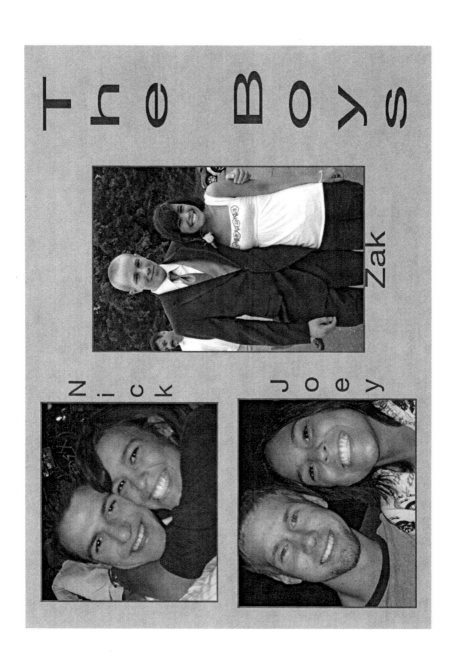

Zak

Nick

Joey

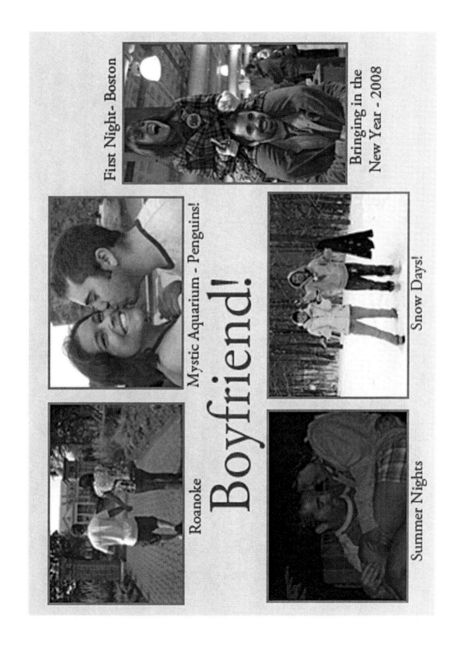

First Night - Boston

Bringing in the
New Year - 2008

Mystic Aquarium - Penguins!

Snow Days!

Roanoke

Boyfriend!

Summer Nights

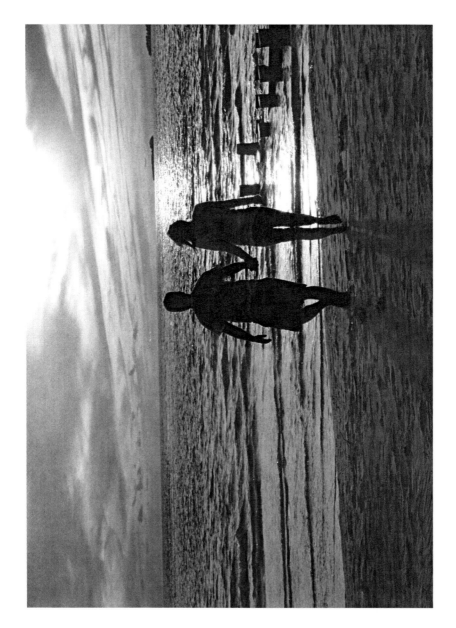

Breinigsville, PA USA
01 March 2010
233368BV00004B/6/P